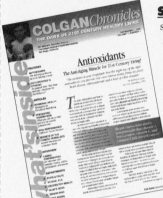

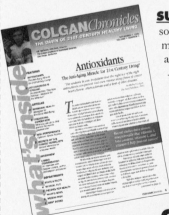

FOR YOU

SUBSCRIBE <u>TO-DAY</u> & GET INFORMED!

YES!
<small>(check one)</small>

☐ I would like a 1 YEAR (8 issues) SUBSCRIPTION for $64. ($88. Cdn)

☐ I would like a 2 YEAR (16 issues) SUBSCRIPTION for $128. ($176. Cdn)

☐ Please send <u>ONE</u> SAMPLE issue for $8. ($11. Cdn) which I understand will be deducted from the total annual subscription rate should I later choose to subscribe (US and Canada only).

(check one)

☐ Please start my subscription with back issues beginning from JANUARY
☐ Please start my subscription with the latest up-coming issue.

NAME _____ TEL ( ) _____

ADDRESS _____

CITY _____ STATE/PROV _____ CODE _____

VISA/MC# _____ EXP _____

☐ Check enclosed to: APPLE PUBLISHING (amount) $ _____

COLGANChronicles is published by: **APPLE PUBLISHING** 4936 Lake Terrell Rd., Ferndale, WA USA 98248
IN CANADA: 220 East 59th Ave, Vancouver, BC V5X 1X9 • ISSN #1206–2863 • Cdn GST#R897232880
Cdn Residents add 7% GST/WA Residents add Sales Tax • Overseas add $25./yr (US Funds) • 4–6 weeks for delivery

---

FOR A FRIEND

SUBSCRIBE <u>TO-DAY</u> & GET INFORMED!

YES!
<small>(check one)</small>

☐ I would like a 1 YEAR (8 issues) SUBSCRIPTION for $64. ($88. Cdn)

☐ I would like a 2 YEAR (16 issues) SUBSCRIPTION for $128. ($176. Cdn)

☐ Please send <u>ONE</u> SAMPLE issue for $8. ($11. Cdn) which I understand will be deducted from the total annual subscription rate should I later choose to subscribe (US and Canada only).

(check one)

☐ Please start my subscription with back issues beginning from JANUARY
☐ Please start my subscription with the latest up-coming issue.

NAME _____ TEL ( ) _____

ADDRESS _____

CITY _____ STATE/PROV _____ CODE _____

VISA/MC# _____ EXP _____

☐ Check enclosed to: APPLE PUBLISHING (amount) $ _____

COLGANChronicles is published by: **APPLE PUBLISHING** 4936 Lake Terrell Rd., Ferndale, WA USA 98248
IN CANADA: 220 East 59th Ave, Vancouver, BC V5X 1X9 • ISSN #1206–2863 • Cdn GST#R897232880
Cdn Residents add 7% GST/WA Residents add Sales Tax • Overseas add $25./yr (US Funds) • 4–6 weeks for delivery

hormonal HEALTH

Dr. Michael COLGAN

NUTRITIONAL AND HORMONAL STRATEGIES FOR EMOTIONAL WELL-BEING & INTELLECTUAL LONGEVITY

Apple Publishing
Vancouver, British Columbia
Canada 1996

For information contact: Apple Publishing, 220 East 59th Avenue, Vancouver, British Columbia, Canada V5X 1X9
Tel (604) 325-2888 • Fax (604) 322-6978

FIRST EDITION

Canadian Cataloguing in Publication Data

Colgan, Michael, 1939–
    Hormonal health : nutritional & hormonal strategies for emotional well-being and intellectual longevity

Includes bibliographical references and index,
ISBN 0-9695272-7-6

    1. Hormones, Sex. 2. Sex (Biology)--Nutritional aspects. I. Title.

RM294.C64 1996   613.9'5   C96-900272-6

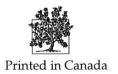

Printed in Canada

To Michael, Dick, Rhys,
Stuart, James,
and my Lesley,
who lent me their courage
when mine was lacking

Also by Dr. Michael Colgan:

Electrodermal Responses
The Training Index
The Power Program
Your Personal Vitamin Profile
Prevent Cancer Now
Optimum Sports Nutrition
The New Nutrition: Medicine for the Millennium
Sexual Potency

Forewords

*"Stop whatever you're doing and read **"Hormonal Health."** Dr. Colgan's amazing new book is vital to your health. He has been a leader in nutritional research for 20 years. Now he has pioneered a new health horizon."*

> Dr. Richard Passwater
> Director of Research
> Solgar Vitamin Co.

*"Oh, have we been waiting for this book. In **Hormonal Health** Michael Colgan gives you everything you need for a new level of extended healthy life. Far ahead of his time, Dr. Colgan draws together the science and medicine of many diverse fields into the first real nutritional, hormonal and lifestyle guide to inhibit aging.*

Crammed with wicked wit and wisdom, irreverent and impertinent, his clear, concise and easily understandable writing is a treat. Ramrod straight he goes for the jugular of science every time, each conclusion strapped tight to impeccable medical references. And the man himself is a living example of everything he advocates"

> Ben Weider, PhD
> President, International Federation of Bodybuilders

"One of the anointed authorities on health and healing recently enumerated what allopathic medicine can and cannot do. Chronic degenerative diseases including hormonal imbalances is one of the "cannot" areas. Dr. Michael Colgan, one of the most eloquent nutrition experts of our time, has addressed the endocrine system in a blockbuster guide, **Hormonal Health***. This book is a must for every health conscious consumer seeking to understand the "big picture" of which hormones are the key. It is going to be my reference guide and that of my co-host, Donald Carrow, M.D., Talk Radio's Medical Maverick."*

    Deborah A. Ray, M.T.

    Host, Radio Station "Here's To Your Health!"

"Like a prophet in the wilderness, Dr. Colgan cries out to all who will listen. For those who will follow his leadings (and heed his warnings) the richness of a vibrant health span lay before you. But woe be unto those who tarry until mainstream medicine begrudgingly yields to the prophetic fulfillment."

    Doug Benbow

    USA Masters Natural Bodybuilding Champion

    Technical advisor and model for Soloflex Inc.

"Dr. Michael Colgan through the years has been one of our best scientific researchers to have presented information to the thousands of professionals who attend our international seminars. We originally selected Dr. Colgan as a speaker as a result of his well written and well documented research and published works we had studied as well as marketed in our international professional bookstore. His most recent book, **Hormonal Health**, is another great tribute to his excellent research and his easily readable literary style. One of the most notable aspects of Dr. Colgan's approach in **Hormonal Health**, as well as his previous works, is that all of his information is validated and supported by accepted research protocols. You just can't go wrong following Dr. Colgan's recommendations. As important as the hormonal system is to normal functioning of the human body in health and disease, we would encourage everyone to obtain, read, and utilize the information in this excellent book."

Dr. W. Karl Parker
COO, Parker Chiropractic, Dallas.

"Becoming acquainted with the interaction and influence of hormones has been of the most powerful lessons for me in learning how to empower others to transform their physiques. After reading your newest work, **Hormonal Health**, I realized how limited my scope of knowledge in the area truly was. Again, Dr. Colgan, you've opened new doors for me, and I feel it is the responsibility of the health and fitness industries to spread the invaluable information you continue to uncover and share. Amidst the abundance of misinformation and deception in the health related fields, it's always reassuring to know there is a steadfast source of 'the real story'."

Phil Kaplan
Radio Program
International Fitness Consultant
Author, **Mind & Muscle, Fitness For All of You**.

"It has been my pleasure to know Dr. Colgan and use his information for over 10 years. I really appreciate the fact that he is a leader in putting out current information on topics that haven't been explored as well as they should. This is very important to the users and merchandisers of nutritional supplements. His unique composite of scientific background and clinical experience give great value to his work. In addition he references his works well. I have worked in this field for over 25 years and these works are invaluable. Authors who do these works do as much to improve the health of their fellow man as the researchers who do the work."

Joseph M. Bassett
Past President
of National Nutritional Foods Association.

"Michael Colgan does it again - his ability to bring clarity to a complicated subject is evidenced in **Hormonal Health***. Dr. Colgan's previous book,* **Optimum Sports Nutrition***, has become a 'Bible' in the field of sports nutrition. Dr. Colgan has the rare ability to deliver understandable, usable, up-to-date information to a field where rampant misinformation is the standard. Any book written by Colgan is a must in my library. His wit and sense of humor make dry subjects enjoyable and entertaining."*

Dr. Ann de Wees Allen
M² Corporation.

"As a long time admirer of the professionalism and straight forwardness of Dr. Colgan's work, I highly recommend this book to everyone who is concerned as to their state of mental and physical well being."

Jim Heflin, President
Beverly International Nutrition.

*"**Hormonal Health** is jam packed with unique and provocative hypotheses which are backed up by Dr. Colgan's vast research. He distills the most sophisticated information into language that is easily understood. Then Dr. Colgan adds his unique point of view spiced with his cutting wit. Once again, Dr. Colgan, you have challenged us all with this hard hitting book."*

Richie Gerber, B.A., L.N.C.
Radio program
Co-owner Bread of Life Natural Foods
Supermarkets.

*"Dr. Colgan pulls no punches and isn't afraid to call it like he sees it. We need more advocates like him to protect against abuses in the medical and drug industries. Any consumer in the health care field (aren't we all?) needs to carefully consider the facts in **Hormonal Health**."*

Joe Weider, President
Weider Health & Fitness

*"**Hormonal Health** will be required reading for those in our technical department as well as all representatives dealing with consumers and health food stores. I advise everyone in the industry to read it. Dr. Colgan continues to present well documented information vital to those persons interested in taking responsibility for their own health in our current health care system. If you are interested in raising the quality, as well as increasing the length of your life, read his books."*

Tim Avila
R&D Coordinator
Unipro

"Congratulations, Dr. Colgan, on your new book, **Hormonal Health**! *It is precise, shocking and thought provoking! It should be read by all, especially the female patient, who is interested in good health and the prevention of cancer. Dr. Colgan is a research scientist who knows no fear in seeking out the truth. Again, congratulations on a job well done."*

Donald R. Whitaker, D.O.
Host of TBN, TV "Calling Dr. Whitaker", Dallas.

"Dr. Colgan is a brilliant pioneer in our quest for wellness and prevention, while others focus on illness and cure. His research signals the dawn of a new era in self-awareness and management of human physiology in a world where change is accelerating in fast forward. Read and discover the power within!"

Denis Waitley, Ph.D., Author
"Psychology of Winning"

"Dr. Colgan's wonderful books and articles in New Zealand Fitness magazine are dramatically changing the lifestyles of hundreds of thousands of New Zealanders. This definitely includes our family."

Phillip & Dr. Jackie Mills, Owners
Les Mills World of Fitness
New Zealand

Dr. Colgan has done it again. **Hormonal Health** *tells the real story with no punches pulled about how to straighten out your hormones. It exposes how endogenous hormones become deranged, how exogenous hormones have been used inapproriately, and best of all how to make them right. This book will do for your health what his* **Optimum Sports Nutrition** *did for your muscles.*

Dr. Luke Bucci
Vice President of Research
Weider Nutrition Group

x

"Thank you Dr. Colgan for this hormonal awakening that has traditionally been a hormonal nightmare.

Dr. Colgan has the tenacity and strength that it takes to look at the 'traditional' medical world and ask why? Even more powerful than that... he finds natural alternatives to chemical medicine and teaches us to ask, Why Not? **Hormonal Health** *will revolutionize the way we treat our bodies, our mind and our health. Balance your chemistry... Balance your life!"*

Victoria Johnson
TV Host, Author, Fitness Video Celebrity

"Another great work on a most controversial and critical health issue from one of the nation's premiere authorities on nutrition. **Hormonal Health** *boldly presents and lays waste to the myths and misinformation that threaten our physical, intellectual and emotional health. Bravo, Dr. Colgan."*

Myron W. Wentz, Founder and Chairman of the Board
of Gull Laboratories Inc. and USANA Inc.

Acknowledgments

My wonderful staff and colleagues gave me the impetus to write this book. They urged me to show you the evidence that hormonal health is the key to vitality and longevity. They prompted me to tell you how this most important aspect of health care, especially women's health care, has been grossly mismanaged. They helped me beyond measure to be the herald of the coming revolution in medicine. My thanks to Jeanne Soper, Dawn Gentry, Stephanie Rudy, Mary O'Hara, Gurli Raaberg, Pat Roemer, Andrea Pruitt, Erica Worke, and most of all my wife and fellow scientist Lesley, and all those who have written forewords herein.

Introduction

For the past 22 years I have taught university courses and carried out laboratory and field research on nutritional, hormonal and lifestyle influences on human performance and longevity. I work also as a clinical consultant, and have formulated individual programs for thousands of athletes, and patients referred to me by their physicians. So I am able to view the scientific data both as a scientist, and with the less jaundiced eye of a clinician.

This book analyses the overwhelming evidence from government documents and peer-reviewed research, that medical management of hormonal health lags far behind our scientific knowledge. This lag, coupled with commercial greed, has prevented physicians from gaining the information and thus delivering the health care that can inhibit many of the degenerative diseases of aging.

For the first time in history, medical science has gained sufficient knowledge of human functioning, to understand how the hormonal cascade that flows from your brain, controls the structure of your body, your energy, your emotions, even how well you can think. By simple maintenance of your hormonal system, using nutrients and non-toxic amounts of certain hormones and other compounds, it is now possible to extend healthy human life by at least 30 years.

At the Colgan Institute we have been using the evidence, of hormonal maintenance since 1982, to formulate our **Hormonal Health Program**. Today, in 1996, I am satisfied that the science has advanced sufficiently to present the basic principles in a book for the public.

One book, however, can cover only a tiny fraction of the evidence. I have done my best to ensure it is a true and representative fraction. Even so, this work is on the cutting edge of science and I am a scientist not a physician. I urge you therefore, to examine the medical references given, and to take them to your physician. It is their exclusive function to give you medical advice. If you adopt anything in this book without first gaining your physician's approval, you do so upon your own choice and risk.

There are profound biochemical differences between individuals that can negate any conclusion drawn from the averages that result from scientific studies of groups. Only your physician can obtain the correct testing and other information required to estimate the unique needs of your individual physiology.

Nevertheless, I am satisfied that the science reviewed herein, when properly used under medical advice, will bring about revolutionary changes in health care, as important as those that followed the work of Pasteur. It is towards this end that I dedicate my work.

Michael Colgan
San Diego
March 1996

Contents

Chapters

Chemical Castration

Put three bulls in with your herd and they will beat each other half to death in testosterone-spiked fights for sexual dominance. Stallions have to be kept apart too. Some riding stables don't want stallions on the premises, because even their smell scares the geldings, and drives the mares crazy. The majority of male horses are gelded early, so they will ignore sex, lose their natural aggression, and become quiet enough to handle.

Eastern potentates played this game for thousands of years, and still do. Castrating young soldiers into eunuchs makes them reliably docile work horses, and totally uninterested in the ladies. They whine and bitch a lot, but they lack the spunk to revolt.

Millions of American men and women suffer the same fate today. Castration is also widespread in Canada, Great Britain, Europe, Australia, and New Zealand. But our castration is hidden, disguised by the trappings of modern life. As you will see, hundreds of medical drugs, unnecessary surgery, witches' brews of pollutants, nutritional deficiencies, and social forces conspire today to make us both docile and impotent.

The Fall Of The West

Our forefathers were potent. The pioneers were tough, courageous, aggressive. That's how a tiny few men and women on horseback were able to tame ferocious countries like America, India, Africa, and Australia. But today most wranglers ride geldings. Why? Because the impotence of the horse matches the impotence of the rider.

In our panty-waist modern life, stallions are too feisty for any but the strongest men. John Wayne and the Magnificent Seven aside, the American cowboy image of strength, courage, and real man spunk, provides a perfect parable of what is happening to our potency. Most of the fearless Hollywood horsemen riding off into the sunset, are foppish pretenders on impotent steeds.

The stuff of bulls, stallions, and real men and women is the strongest drive in all the animal kingdom. In her typical economy, Nature also uses the mechanisms of this reproductive urge to drive confidence, courage, strength, well-being, leadership and love. As sexual potency wanes, a woman loses more than her libido, a man becomes spineless in more than his penis. They lose the very essence that drives the human spirit.

Yet instead of respecting it, nurturing it, learning to enhance it, America and much of the rest of Western Society, seem hell bent on destroying the stuff that made our forefathers great. Chemical castration is rapidly creating impotent nations of wimps.

Eunuchs Galore

The huge increase in American impotence serves as a model of what is happening in other countries. It so concerns the medical community, that in December 1992 the National Institutes of Health, the National Institute of Diabetes, and the National Institute on Aging convened a giant conference. After churning through thousands of research papers, they estimated that completely impotent American males number between 10 and 20 million. That's about a quarter of the adult male population, one man in every four.[1]

In the 1940's only *half* that proportion of males was impotent, about one man in eight.[1] Childless couples were rare. Now over five million American couples are being treated for inability to have children. Men hate to admit it, but much of the problem lies with them.

Medical Malarky

The increase in male impotence is even worse when you consider the huge advances in medical science over the last 50 years. It amazes me that a society with sufficient scientific expertise to clone human embryos,[2] has failed to develop any system to maintain our twin contemporary gods of youth and potency. Rather than improving potency, our health-care system has doubled the rate of impotence and decimated our ability to bear children. Corrupt and misguided health policies have developed thousands of medical drugs, man-made toxins, nutritional deficits, and lifestyle practices that progressively destroy potency. Sounds too fantastic? Read on, I document every one of these claims with impeccable studies from the medical literature.

The typical medical response to this vast problem, resembles the antics of medieval nincompoops who tied feathers to their arms to imitate the appearance of birds in vain attempts to fly. Many physicians try to restore the stuff that makes men men, by imitating its outward appearance. Americans spend multi-millions every year on primitive plastic props, or crude pump-up implants, to hoist the ailing penis aloft, or injectable drugs that turn it temporarily as rigid and senseless as a frankfurter in the freezer.[3]

Midst a fanfare of media praise, the US Food and Drug Administration has just approved another drug **alprostadil** (Caverject) for injection into the penis to create imitation erections.[4] Britain and most of Europe have used it for years. Penile tomfoolery!

For women, the typical medical response is even worse. Until recently, the sexually potent woman was considered somehow immoral, and certainly not to be encouraged or enhanced by medical means.[5] Let's see how this ludicrous state of affairs came about, because once you understand the mechanisms, remaining hormonally healthy and enhancing that power, is a gift you will cherish for life.

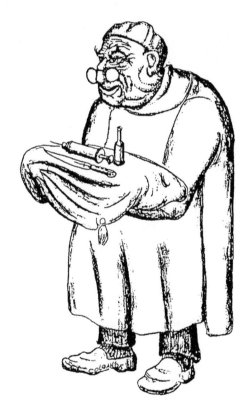

Figure 1. The Castrator's apprentice (after Daumier).

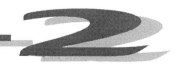

Female Repression

The **Kinsey Report**, presented the first scientific analysis of female sexuality in 1953. Contrary to traditional beliefs, it showed that the majority of women experience intense sexual desire, and sexual excitement, and can achieve orgasm. It even claimed that some 15% of women enjoy multiple orgasms.[1] The general media reaction varied from skepticism to moral outrage. The social climate of the time was not ready for hormonally potent women.[2,3]

Along with the general trend towards social emancipation of women, acceptance had grown by the time William Masters and Virginia Johnson began using electrodes attached to the vagina to record female orgasms in the 1960s.[4] But Puritan morality still held sway, and for much of America, Great Britain, and Europe, a woman's sexuality concerned marital service to her husband. Attempts to enhance sexual and hormonal health, or even to work out the mechanisms, were seen as pandering to the unholy hedonism of Pagan rituals.

Today science has prevailed, and we know that women have the same physiological potential for sexual and hormonal potency as men.[4] Western society is slowly accepting that the hormonal suppression of women is an uncivilized remnant of medieval morality. Science has shown that male and female hormonal potency are both driven by the same physiological mechanisms. World expert, Professor Helen Singer Kaplan, Director of the Human Sexuality Program at Cornell University, keeps a running review of all major studies. There is no longer any doubt that both male and female libido and emotions depend on the same biochemical activity of certain nerve circuits in the brain.

One essential component for these areas to function properly is a critical level of the hormone **testosterone**. Yes, testosterone is not only the stuff of bulls, stallions, and real men, but women too. Men need more testosterone than women, but if it drops below the gender-required level in either sex, libido declines to a whimper.[5] And so do confidence, well-being, love, and zest for life.

Scientists now accept that testosterone fires not only male and female sexual desire, but also controls many other attributes of potency in both sexes.[4] But just as the repressive morality of yesteryear was yielding to science, along came the medicine men to spoil it.

Medical Sexual Repression

The oral contraceptive pill was introduced in 1959. Ask most women today, and they still cannot tell you how it works. Almost all forms of the pill work by suppression of female output of **gonadotropins**, hormones that stimulate sexual functions. The 1995 **Physicians Desk Reference** repeats this statement more than 50 times between pages 615 and 2748.[6]

Some of your most important gonadotropins are those that stimulate manufacture of testosterone. In suppressing gonadotropins to prevent conception, the pill also suppresses testosterone as a side-effect. Suppressed along with it are all the other attributes of your sexual potency, including libido, confidence, courage, and general well-being.[7]

Very few of the more than 14,000 women who have come to the Colgan Institute for nutritional analyses, had been told by their physicians of these side-effects of the pill. Most are told the opposite, that the relief from the anxiety of becoming pregnant offered by the Pill, will increase sexuality. As you will see, that view is contrary to the evidence.[8]

Restrictive religious morality used to keep many women docile and sexually repressed by the same mechanism. Studies show that women brought up to believe that sexuality should be restricted to marriage and childbearing, have lower testosterone levels than those with more liberal attitudes.[7]

Just when the religious norms were changing to become more consistent with the new roles of women in today's world, moral suppression of sexuality was replaced by much more insidious and harmful chemical repression, by the contraceptive pill.

Continuation of this hormonal suppression lifelong is now almost routine, even continuing after menopause, as incorrect estrogen replacement therapy. It is an indictment of health-care systems throughout the Western world, that nearly half of all women have their hormonal health progressively damaged by steroid hormones for most of their adult lives. But don't fret. True hormonal emancipation of women is coming fast.

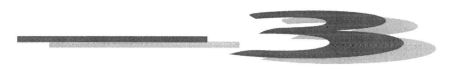

All In Your Head

Recent science shows that the cascade of hormones from your pituitary gland, depends on the orchestrated interactions of dozens of brain chemicals. To understand hormonal health, first we have to take a peek at your brainworks.

The brain has four hollow chambers inside called **ventricles**, filled with cerebrospinal fluid. The top three combine into the three-dimensional shape shown in Figure 2, a bit like the Starship Enterprise. The **hypothalamus** which, as you will see, is the nerve center for control of sex hormones and for libido, straddles part of the front and side walls of the third ventricle. See your hypothalamus as the bridge of the Enterprise, the command center for the chemistry of all your emotional reactions. Below it, the **substantia nigra** is the engine room, sending power signals all over the ship.

The other areas responsible for your hormonal potency, form a good part of the inner walls and floor of the two lateral ventricles. They run back from your temples to past your ears on each side of the brain, with two bulbs running forward again to about ear level. Collectively these areas around the ventricles are called the **striatum** (striped body), or **striatal cortex**.[1]

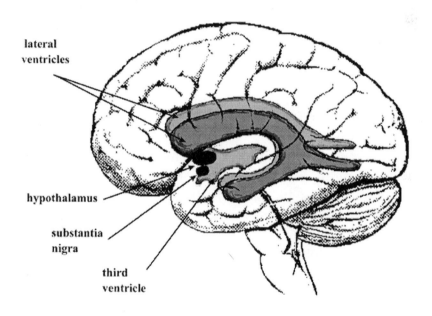

lateral
ventricles

hypothalamus

substantia
nigra

third
ventricle

Figure 2. Three-dimensional shape of top three ventricles in the brain.

All your hormonal brainworks are very old. They were present in the brains of our animal ancestors when they first crawled out of the primieval swamps. Some researchers claim that without the potent drive created by your sex hormones, these primitive creatures would never have made it, and we wouldn't be here today.

One of my TV clients tells me that many of the ideas for starships and aliens come from studying these ancient brain structures. And the programs get their huge followings of fans partly because they "fit" so well with the threads of evolution that bind the human psyche. Maybe so, but remember, its just an analogy. Your brain is far more complex than any starship.

"Captain To Engine Room . . . ."

The main way your brain communicates with itself, so as to work in harmony, is by neural transmission. Different parts of the brain are a bit like starship control systems, each drawing on the available power and contributing unique bursts of information, so that what comes up on the screen of your mind is intelligible, and fits with the power output of your arms, legs, mouth, and other bits. These bursts of information flow electrochemically along nerves, combining and recombining, into the symphony of consciousness, just as the notes of different instruments combine in an orchestra.

As Figure 3 illustrates, each nerve cell has many projections called **dendrites**, which receive information from adjacent cells and carry it to the cell body. Just like a computer chip, the cell body then makes a decision to fire or not to fire. When it does fire, a long projection called an **axon**, carries the information on to the dendrites of the next lot of cells.

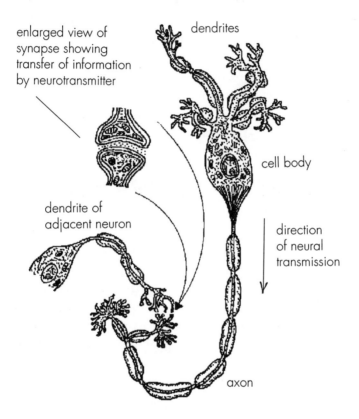

enlarged view of synapse showing transfer of information by neurotransmitter

dendrites

cell body

dendrite of adjacent neuron

direction of neural transmission

axon

Figure 3. Schematic of a nerve cell.

But unlike computer chips, which are all hard-wired together, nerve cells are separated from each other by gaps called **synapses**. Information is carried across the gaps by special chemical transporters called **neurotransmitters**, which flow out of the end of the axon. After the information reaches the neighboring dendrites, the neurotransmitter is sucked up again into the nerve terminal.

That's the *way* it happens. But there's more than one *type* of neurotransmitter. Dozens of different types complement or inhibit each other, to prevent or to facilitate information flow. What gets through depends on the *amounts* of each neurotransmitter present at the synapses of nerves in different parts of the brain. The sum of all the inputs, moment-to-moment, is what you experience as cognition, emotions, and sexuality.

Neurotransmitters Control Hormones

To dodge a mountain of biochemistry, we will oversimplify a bit and confine attention to the main excitatory and inhibitory neurotransmitters in the sexual circuits of your brain, the hypothalamus, substantia nigra, and striatum. The primary excitatory neurotransmitter is **dopamine**. The second excitatory neurotransmitter is **acetylcholine**. The two main inhibitory neurotransmitters are **serotonin and noradrenalin (norepinephrine)**.[2] Maintaining hormonal health means maintaining the balance between these brain chemicals. It's as simple as that - almost.

Different bits of your sexual areas, however, have different functions. The hypothalamus, substantia nigra and bottom or ventral areas of the striatum, are primary for libido and emotion. The upper or dorsal striatum is primary for control of alertness, arousal and orgasm.[3,4] Some strategies to optimize hormonal health affect one area more than another. The ideal strategy is a combination that stimulates everything equally. Before you can arrive at such a nirvana, it pays to know some of the other mechanisms of your sexuality. They are firmly tied to every other aspect of your life.

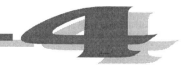

Sex & Emotions

When I was a graduate student, a series of experiments we did in neurophysiology involved implanting rats with tiny electrodes in the **medial preoptic nucleus** of the **hypothalamus**. The hypothalamus of your brain mediates many complex functions, including feelings of pleasure, excitement, anger, anxiety, fear, hunger, thirst and temperature regulation.[1] It also mediates release of the brain hormone cascade that controls the production of sex hormones.[2]

If you send tiny pulsed electrical charges through the electrodes, the preoptic nucleus interprets them as activation of libido. This activation puts male rats into a constant state of sexual excitement (and penile erection). Provided with a continuing supply of fresh females, they engage in an orgy of sexual intercourse, ignoring food, sleep, and comfort until they keel over from exhaustion.

The rat is a simple creature, but humans and monkeys have similar areas in the hypothalamus, as shown in Figure 4. And electrical stimulation of the preoptic area readily produces sexual arousal and penile erection in monkeys.[3]

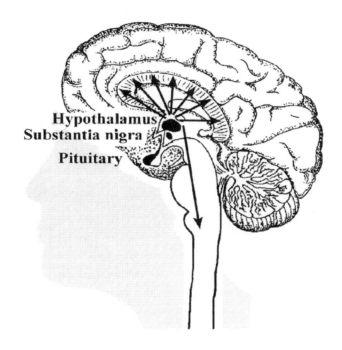

Figure 4. Section through human brain showing areas that mediate libido.

It's a bit difficult to get healthy humans to volunteer for needle electrodes implanted in their brains. But a number of human studies using these electrodes to relieve intractable depression, show that men can be sexually aroused by the same hypothalamic stimulation that fires rats and monkeys.[1]

In some cases the electrodes are attached to a switch box, permitting the patient to self-stimulate. In my lectures, I show a film of a man, who spent most of his days in deep depression, sitting motionless in a chair. An implant that allowed self-stimulation of various areas of the hypothalamus, activated his libido, and associated feelings of well-being and confidence, every time he pressed a button on a box attached to his belt. This electrical stimulation did the job so well, it transformed him into a raunchy nightclub comedian, good enough to be paid for his act. **There is no doubt that the preoptic nucleus, and other areas of the hypothalamus, are mediators of human libido.**[1]

Testosterone and Libido

In the absence of an electrode, stuck into your brain to fire libido, how does it work? To find out we have had to dip into a little biochemistry. Bear with me, you don't have to be a rocket scientist to follow it. And follow it you should, because libido is the base of hormonal health. Without it, much of life is reduced to mere mechanical twitch and whimper.

It's no surprise that the hypothalamus, which mediates your libido, also controls the manufacture of all your sex hormones, even though the manufacturing organs are in parts of the body remote from your brain. The **arcuate nucleus** of the hypothalamus secretes a brain hormone called **gonadotropin-releasing hormone (GRH)**. This hormone trickles down into the anterior (front) lobe of the pituitary gland, the pea-sized blob hanging out of your brain, on a stalk, a couple of inches behind your nose. It's a busy blob.

In both males and females, the anterior or front of the pituitary manufactures all sorts of hormones every day of your life. In this chapter we will cover only three that are intimately involved with libido. They are shown in Figure 5.

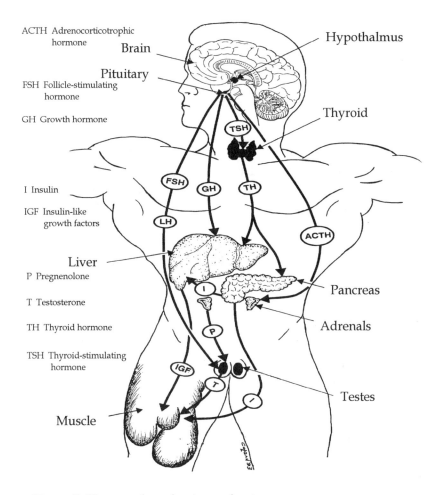

Figure 5. Hormonal mechanisms of potency.

The first is **luteinizing hormone**. Under the influence of GRH, your pituitary gland releases luteinizing hormone which flows to the testicles in males, where it stimulates special structures called **Leydig cells** to produce testosterone. Healthy, potent men make about 7 mg of testosterone per day.[4] That's plenty to flow throughout the body and brain to maintain male masculinity, and hormonal potency.

In females, luteinizing hormone flows to the ovaries and to the adrenal glands, where it also stimulates testosterone production. Healthy, potent women make about 0.3 mg of testosterone per day in the ovaries, the adrenals, and various other parts of the body.

It used to be a puzzle why females produce testosterone at all. Then studies showed that the hormone is as essential for a woman's hormonal health as it is for a man's. **We know now that testosterone is a primary stimulant of the hypothalamus and other brain areas that activates both male and female libido.**[5,6]

Along with luteinizing hormone, the anterior pituitary in both sexes also secretes **follicle-stimulating hormone (FSH).** In women, FSH is vital to the menstrual cycle and reproduction. In men, it triggers the **Sertoli cells** of the testicles to make sperm. So it is essential part of overall potency. But as far as we know, FSH has little effect on libido, or emotions.

Thyroid and Libido

With all the evidence linking testosterone and libido, the effects of **thyroid hormones** are sadly neglected, even in medical texts. Big mistake. As I review elsewhere,[4] keeping the thyroid in balance is essential to the balance of many other hormones and systems throughout your body.

Thyroid hormone levels are controlled by output of another hormone from the hypothalamus, **thyrotropin-releasing hormone** (see Figure 5). It flows to the anterior pituitary to cause release of **thyroid-stimulating hormone (TSH)** which, in turn, stimulates the thyroid gland at the base of your neck to produce thyroid hormones. As you might guess from this complex series of checks and balances, thyroid hormones have powerful effects.

Yet synthetic thyroid is commonly believed to be relatively innocuous, and seems to be used in America almost as freely as aspirin. We find that numerous athletes, models, and celebrities who come to the Colgan Institute for nutrition programs, have normal thyroid function, but have been prescribed thyroid pills or use them without prescription. Reasons range from losing bodyfat to a general pick-me-up.

More like a general knock-you-down. Studies show without a doubt, that excess serum levels of thyroid (hyperthyroidism) reduce libido and positive emotions to a whimper.[7]

Excess thyroid is also catabolic (destructive) to most body tissues. That's why some folk use it to lose fat. But it is equally destructive to muscle.[8] As we will see in later chapters, maintaining muscle is one of the essential strategies for all aspects of hormonal health. So taking thyroid pills, except in the case of a well-documented thyroid deficiency, delivers a triple-whammy to your muscles, libido and well-being.

Low thyroid (hypothyroidism) is just as bad. When you have insufficient thyroid to help drive your insulin metabolism, multiple body functions go crazy.[9] Low thyroid not only causes lethargy and exhaustion, it also reduces testosterone levels.[10] And you know by now that reduced testosterone whacks your libido. Don't fret. We cover strategies to keep your thyroid healthy in the chapters on nutrition.

Prolactin and Libido

The final hormone that profoundly affects libido is **prolactin**, the milk-producing hormone that enables women to breastfeed. Males also produce prolactin. In both sexes it is released by the anterior pituitary.

Unlike most other pituitary hormones, control of the prolactin is mainly inhibitory. Prolactin output is restricted by release of the neurotransmitter dopamine from the arcuate nucleus of the hypothalamus.[11] That's the same blob of brain that stimulates secretion of luteinizing hormone to drive testosterone production. If the flow of dopamine declines, prolactin secretion hits the roof, and testosterone levels hit the floor. The astute reader will appreciate Nature's design in thus neatly reducing libido while women are breastfeeding.

In men, excess prolactin has the same detrimental effects on testosterone, and thereby on libido. But that's not part of Nature's design for health. In males, high prolactin is an indicator of brain disorder.

Reduced hypothalamic dopamine also inhibits libido directly. Recent science shows that brain areas that drive your libido and emotions, require healthy levels of both testosterone and dopamine for normal function.[12]

The three main causes of excess prolactin production are hypothyroidism, which we discussed above, prescription drugs, discussed in later chapters, and -- stress. Stress activates numerous subjective feelings, from loss of well-being and loss of confidence, through anxiety, fear, anger, and hate. All negative emotions have profound adverse effects on hormonal health.

Libido and Aging

Various studies of male libido show a maximum strength at about age 17-20 with a slow decline to about age 45-50. About age 50, enough men show a sharp decline in libido, to prompt researchers to create the notion of **viripause**, akin to the female menopause. Some of these men do show abnormally low testosterone levels, without any other signs of illness, which suggests there may be a grain of truth to male menopause. In these individuals, restoring testosterone levels to normal also restores libido and well-being.[13]

Trouble is, all studies to date of aging, sex and emotion have failed to separate out men who are healthy in all the bodily systems important to sexuality. The best yet is by Dr. Raul Schiavi and colleagues at Mt. Sinai School of Medicine in New York.[14] Their select sample of men aged 45-74, had no diseases or disorders likely to impair sexuality. They were not more than 20% overweight, and didn't take drugs. Results still showed that libido declined with age.

But even this study failed to select the sample for one variable that is critical to hormonal health - maintenance of youthful muscle mass. With usual aging, even apparently healthy men, lose one-quarter of their muscle mass between ages 20 and 80.[15] So it's likely that Schiavi's sample were short on muscle. As we will see in a later chapter, if you fail to keep sufficient muscle, decline of many bodily functions, including sex hormones and libido, is inevitable.

All major surveys, from Kinsey[16,17] through the Baltimore Gerontology Center Study,[18] show highly variable levels of libido with age. Some older men exhibit stronger libido than some young men and vice-versa. Some old men report no change in libido throughout life. So it is likely that most losses of male libido found with age, are more a sign of degeneration than passing of the years.

In females, however, there are definite age changes in libido. Young women do not reach peak libido until age 35-40. Even after menopause, the ovaries and adrenal glands of most women continue to produce some testosterone.

Nevertheless, at Cornell Medical Center in New York, Dr. Helen Singer Kaplan has found that at least 15-20% of postmenopausal women show low testosterone levels and associated loss of libido and zest for life. In many of these women, low-dose testosterone replacement therapy promptly restores potency.[19]

Loss of libido is especially likely in women whose menopause is surgically induced. But we will come to the horrors of hysterectomy in a later chapter. Before that, we have to examine the rest of hormonal health, including the puzzles of orgasm, and the links between these physiological responses and emotional and intellectual well-being.

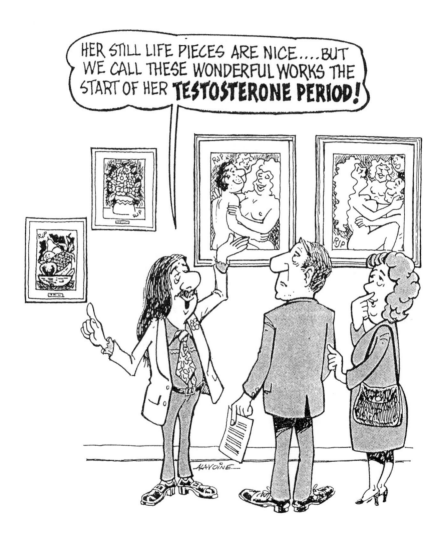

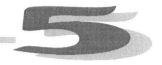

Orgasm

The physiological mechanism of orgasm is identical for men and women. Orgasmic sensation is produced by rhythmic contractions of the **ischiocavernosii** and **bulbocavernosii** muscles. In males, these muscles are at the base of the penis. In females, they are inside and around the vaginal opening. As soon as arousal reaches a certain level, orgasm occurs automatically, a magnificent symphony of neural, hormonal, and muscular reactions.

Women, however, have much greater difficulty reaching this state than men. The authoritative new survey, **Sex in America**, done at the University of Chicago, National Opinion Research Center, shows that less than one-third of American women always have orgasm during sex. One woman in five was unable to achieve orgasm in the past year. In contrast, three-quarters of American men always achieve orgasm.[1] A sad state of affairs, because healthy subjects of both sexes rate orgasm among the most euphoric of human experiences.

Male Orgasm

The three aspects of orgasm most folk want to improve are **duration, frequency,** and **intensity**. In men, the physiological purpose of orgasmic contractions is to propel semen forcefully from the penis. So the number of contractions, and thus, the duration of orgasm, depends largely on the volume of available ejaculate.[2] Very potent men have enough for 10-12 contractions each lasting up to a second.

A refractory period follows male orgasm, that is a time during which no further orgasms can occur. Though scientists don't know for sure, it's likely that length of the refractory period, and therefore the maximum frequency of orgasm, depends on how long it takes for ejaculate to build up again.

Most of the fluid portion of ejaculate comes from the prostate gland. With usual aging the prostate overgrows, and ejaculate volume and manufacture diminishes. The duration of orgasms diminishes accordingly. The refractory period also lengthens, from minutes at age 20, to as much as 48 hours by age 70, sharply curtailing orgasm frequency.[3]

So, to maintain male orgasmic capacity it's vital to maintain a healthy prostate. Though it isn't difficult to do so, most men fail miserably. Prostate problems are so common after age 40, that I deal with how to correct them, in a separate chapter ahead.

Intensity of male orgasm is not dependent on ejaculate. Rather it is a complex interaction of neural and hormonal reactions. Along with hormonal potency, **The Hormonal Health Program** ahead, is widely praised by users as a boost to orgasmic intensity.

Female Orgasm

In female orgasm the same muscles contract with the same frequency as in men.[2] But contractions are not limited by ejaculate because there is none. So there's no refractory period either, and no decline of orgasmic capacity with aging. Healthy women are capable of intense orgasms lifelong.[2]

Common aging problems that reduce female orgasm, are progressive fragility of vaginal membranes and loss of vaginal lubrication. Because female genitals require a good supply of estrogen for daily maintenance, these problems worsen with menopause. The resulting discomfort and fear of injury limit all sexuality.[3]

You can easily correct vaginal dryness with lubricants. Don't use the commonly advised synthetic petroleum products. Health food stores stock numerous vegetable oil emulsions, usually sold as "body lotions", that nicely simulate vaginal secretions.

You can also correct vaginal fragility by judicious hormone replacement therapy. But use of exogenous hormones affects not only orgasm, but all aspects of sexual potency. So I cover this complex subject in separate chapters ahead.

Regular intercourse is also important to maintain vaginal tone and membrane condition. Many women do not appreciate that abstinence rapidly reduces capacity for orgasm.[2] Use it or lose it. Although female masturbation is still stigmatized in Western Society, in the absence of a sexual partner, it is sensible preventive maintenance.

Religious Repression

Doyenne of sexuality, Helen Singer Kaplan, also indicts some religious teachings with suppression of female orgasm.[3] Raised as a Catholic, I remember well myself being subjected to crippling anti-sexual dogma. At puberty I was ashamed of my sexuality and constantly guilty about my libido, and about the masturbation that relieved it. But being male, I had no problem achieving orgasm.

Women are more subject to these repressive social influences than men because, as we have seen, female sexuality is strongly linked to environmental circumstances and physical and mental ease. Thus their route to orgasm is more delicate, more easily disrupted. In the prestigious **Sex In America** survey, Catholic women were the least likely of the religious groups studied to achieve orgasm.[1] In other studies, women raised to restrict their sexuality to marriage and reproduction show reduced levels of the all important hormone testosterone.[4] Esther Rome, co-author of the famous book **Our Bodies, Ourselves**, concludes that social and cultural norms that ignore the needs of women are likely the major source of female sexual dysfunction.[5]

Before some self-righteous Christians or "family values" supporters moan that I am undermining moral standards by promoting female orgasm, and, O'Lordy, masturbation, let me stress its importance to the very values they uphold.

Considerable evidence now shows that marital satisfaction for women is strongly linked to sexual intercourse with their husbands that culminates in orgasm.[6]

Orgasm and Female Health

Far from being dirty, sinful or immoral, the practices that promote female orgasm are both healthy and natural. Regular manual and oral stimulation of breasts and genitals are just what the doctor ordered to prevent disease and keep these organs in prime condition.

Breast cancer for example, is the second leading cause of cancer death in American women, and is on the rapid rise.[7] One major suspected cause is the accumulation of carcinogenic man-made chemicals in breast tissue, including dioxins, polychlorinated biphenyl's (PCBs) heavy metals, pesticides, and air pollutants. In my book **The New Nutrition**, I review the evidence that accumulation of these toxins increases the risk of breast cancer.[7] Healthy sexual behavior is one good way that women can protect themselves.

Dr. Timothy Murrell, Professor of Medicine at the University of Adelaide, has shown that breast and nipple stimulation, including sucking and squeezing, causes the female body to produce **oxytocin**, a hormone that contracts small muscles in the breast. These contractions squeeze sac-like glands where toxins accumulate, and releases them, both through the nipples and into the blood circulation for excretion. Dr. Murrell's research indicates that regular breast and nipple stimulation has a strong protective effect against breast cancer.[8]   In our fouled world of today, it is sensible preventive maintenance for the female human body.

Oral and manual vaginal stimulation serves similar protective functions. It maintains the tone and condition of the vagina and clitoris against the insidious fragility that occurs with disuse and usual aging. It also maintains a woman's ability to excrete the lubricants which facilitate vaginal intercourse.[2]

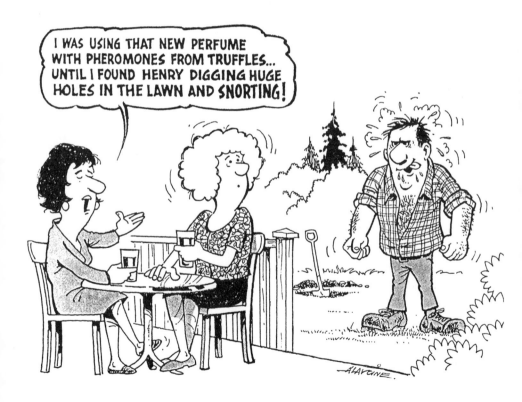

Hormones For Smarts

By now you realize that the brain structures and the hormone cascade that control sexuality, also control many other functions of your body and brain. Startling new research shows that these controls extend even to your ability to reason.

Cognition, intelligence, memory, and sexuality all involve the same brain circuits in the striatal cortex and hypothalamus. The ebb and flow of your sexual hormones influences what you are able to see, hear, and feel, what you are able to understand, and how much you are able to remember. Science is fast coming to realize that these hormones may largely determine the acuteness of our perception of the world, and therefore the sensitivity and the content of our reactions towards each other.

Estrogen and Your Brain

We start with estrogen. Multiple recent studies show that estrogen enhances a woman's sexual and emotional arousal by sensitizing her vision, hearing, smell, taste and touch.[1] Now we are discovering that estrogen's influence extends even to your most secret thoughts.

Alzheimer's disease provides a good starting point. In the early '80s, numerous researchers showed that the dementia (loss of intelligence and social competence) and memory loss of Alzheimer's, is linked to loss of acetylcholine activity and cholinergic neurons in the **substantia nigra**.[2,3] As you know from Chapter 3, acetylcholine is a crucial brain neurotransmitter for sexuality, and the substantia nigra is one of the main brain areas for sexuality in which it operates.

Also in the early '80s, studies on rats showed that estrogen enhances activity of cholinergic neurons in the preoptic area of the hypothalamus, and its projections from the preoptic area into the cerebral cortex, the "center" for cognition. In rats, this area is about equivalent to your substantia nigra, and the sexual bits of your hypothalamus. Brain activity in these animals increased in a dose-dependent fashion. The bigger the estrogen shot, the greater the brain boost.[4,5]

New studies indicate that estrogen also works on cholinergic neurons in humans. First, it influences messenger RNA (ribonucleic acid) to promote new growth of nerve connections. Second, it triggers gene expression (turns on part of a gene) to stimulate acetylcholine production.[6,7] If estrogen has such power, that it can alter the manufacture of brain structures and neurotransmitters at the basic level of your genetic program, then maintenance of youthful levels of this hormone is indeed an essential strategy for healthy brain function.

Estrogen Boosts Intelligence

Does estrogen also affect cognition? You bet! Let's look at what happens to postmenopausal women. These findings are only just now hitting the medical journals. They are dynamite.

At menopause, estrogen production by human ovaries declines from 250-300 micrograms per day to about 20 micrograms, mostly made in the liver. Cognition declines in concert. Drs. Barbara Sherwin and Diane Kampen at McGill University recruited apparently healthy women aged 55 and over, all of whom had completed menopause at least two years earlier. One group were on estrogen replacement therapy. A second group of women, matched for social and economic factors with the first group, had not used estrogen to correct their menopausal loss. Tests of verbal recall showed that estrogen users had maintained significantly better memories.[8]

Studies by Drs. David Robinson, Jerome Yesavage and colleagues at Stanford University School of Medicine confirm these findings. Using non-senile women aged 55-93, they have shown that estrogen users have significantly better memories for faces and for words.[9]

Barbara Sherwin has also studied **oophorectomized** women (women who have had their ovaries surgically removed).

Those on estrogen replacement therapy are smarter and have better memories.[10]

Critics of this research point out that the women who were taking estrogen may have been smarter in the first place, and that's why they were using the therapy. So the hormone itself had nothing to do with their test scores. Not so. New research by Dr. Uriel Halbreich and colleagues, at the State University of New York at Buffalo, firmly links estrogen to smarts.

Halbreich recruited postmenopausal women who were not taking estrogen, and tested their reaction time, mental alertness, verbal ability, and other cognitive capacities. He also tested a group of healthy young women. The young group did much better than the old group on all the tests. Then he put the old group on estrogen replacement therapy for 60 days and tested them again. They scored significantly better on all tests, some of them posting test scores higher than some of the young women.[11]

Halbreich also showed that test performance was strongly linked to the amount of estrogen in the older women's blood. The higher the estrogen, the better the test scores. Even in young women, studies of memory during the menstrual cycle show that verbal memories are best when estrogen is highest. It's the hormone for sure that maintains your smarts.[12]

Estrogen Deficit Causes Dementia

The clincher to this startling information is Alzheimer's. To explain our current epidemic of this ghastly malady, uninformed media have been trumpeting connections between Alzheimer's and genetic defects. What a lot of cobblers! It's true that genetic defects on chromosome 14 and chromosome 1 are linked to a few cases of early-onset Alzheimer's in succeeding generations of families.[13,14] But about 90% of Alzheimer's cases, and the growing incidence of the disease, has a simpler explanation.

Consider these five facts:

- Alzheimer's disease doesn't start when you are old. The slow brain degeneration, which finally shows itself in dementia and profound memory loss, begins decades earlier, in your 40s.[15]

- Women suffer much more from Alzheimer's than men.[16]

- Women live longer than men, and their lifespan has increased significantly in Western Society over the last 25 years.[17]

- Women lose over 90% of their estrogen at menopause, whether age-induced or surgically induced via hysterectomy. Most men do not show much estrogen decline with aging, because they have sufficient testosterone to convert to estrogen as needed.

- As we have seen, estrogen deficit reduces intelligence and memory.

Let's put the facts together. The menopausal loss of estrogen in women, combined with their increased lifespan, creates a situation in which the slow brain degeneration caused by insufficient estrogen has the added years it takes to progress into dementia.

Testosterone and Cognition

Males, including their brains, have long been believed to run on testosterone. Young men with high testosterone levels for example, have better visuospatial abilities than controls.[18] And, in old men, testosterone treatment enhances scores on the Block Design test of the Weschler Intelligence Scale.[19]

No one knows the mechanisms by which testosterone influences male cognition. But it may well be secondary to estrogen. Male brains have many more estrogen receptors than testosterone receptors, and also have a good supply of the enzyme **aromatase** which converts testosterone to estrogen. At the 1995 Annual Meeting of the Endocrine Society, researchers presented evidence that this conversion occurs continually in the normal male brain.[20]

Further, in those unfortunate males whose estrogen levels decline, for one reason or another, their cognition may decline too. Studies in Sweden show that men in the early stages of Alzheimer's have much lower estrogen levels than healthy controls.[21] High testosterone levels in males may improve cognition simply by providing abundant raw material to convert to estrogen.

The current epidemic of nearly 5,000,000 cases of Alzheimer's disease in America now occupies more than one-third of all nursing home beds.[15] Unless medicine realizes quickly, that maintaining youthful estrogen levels is crucial to brain health, the rapid aging of Western populations will turn that epidemic into the worst disease nightmare ever visited on the human race.

Estrogen Replacement Maintains Brains

If I'm right that estrogen maintains your ability to think, then estrogen replacement therapy should not only help maintain female sexual potency, but should also help protect female brains. If so, estrogen users should have a lower incidence of Alzheimer's.

Based on some case studies in Italy,[22] I first suggested this notion in 1988, and have been waiting ever since for someone to produce controlled evidence. Now we have some. Drs. Annlia Paganini-Hill and Victor Henderson at the University of Southern California School of Medicine in Los Angeles, examined the medical records of women who had died at the retirement community Leisure World in Laguna Hills, California. They found that women who were on estrogen replacement therapy had a much lower incidence of Alzheimer's disease.[23]

Sure, we need more studies to confirm these findings. But they fit so nicely into what we know about brain function, that it would be foolish to wait perhaps another decade for results. The message is clear. Some of the same mechanisms that drive your sexuality also help to maintain your cognitive ability. Estrogen supports these mechanisms by helping to maintain acetylcholine neurotransmission. If women let their estrogen be decimated by hysterectomy or medication, or allow it to decline with the menopause of usual aging, they lose not only much of their potency, but also a big chunk of the smarts required for continued success in life.

Nutrient Brain Boosters

If your estrogen supply has already been interfered with by the medicine men, or if tests show it is declining, or you are already past menopause, **acetyl-l-carnitine** is a potent nutritional strategy to preserve both brain and sexuality. Note well that it is *not* l-carnitine but acetyl-l-carnitine. There is a whole chemical world of difference.

This nutrient amino acid is used by your brain every day to help maintain acetylcholine metabolism. A huge pile of new studies shows that, even in Alzheimer's and some other forms of dementia, acetyl-l-carnitine can restore a great deal of brain function.[24-26]   Although men are less subject to Alzheimer's and most other forms of senility, acetyl-l-carnitine works equally well in male cases. Before the rot starts, it may prevent it entirely.

In amounts of 1000 - 2000mg per day, acetyl-l-carnitine is non-toxic. This level is probably more than sufficient to prevent acetylcholine decline. Especially so, if taken with the spectrum of complimentary nutrients necessary for hormonal health that I review in the nutrition chapter.

At this writing in March 1996, acetyl-l-carnitine is available freely in U.S. health food stores. But pharmaceutical companies who realize its potential have already petitioned the FDA to restrict it. Get your's while you can.

The second nutrient brain booster is **ginkgo biloba**. Since the '70s controlled research has consistently confirmed, that the active substances extracted from this herb improve brain function, by dilating arteries and increasing the supply of oxygen-rich and nutrient-rich blood to the brain.[27,28]

As we will see in the coming chapter on estrogen therapy, estrogen itself helps to protect brain function, not only by maintaining acetylcholine function, but also by increasing blood flow. Ginkgo, however, does not interact with estrogen and does the job nicely by itself. Though it is non-toxic in any sensible dose, ginkgo can provide such a brain boost that it should be taken only in the morning. Taken later in the day it can cause insomnia.

Weak ginkgo preparations infest the health marketplace. Buy only those that guarantee they are standardized for 24% flavonoid glycosides plus 6%-8% terpene lactones, and 7%-10% proanthocyanidins. The Life Extension Foundation in Florida sells a reliable brand.

Hormone Brain Boosters

The second strategy for you to maintain both hormonal potency and cognition, depends on whether you have menstrual cycles. If you are producing your own estrogen, then don't allow any medicine man to mess with it. And don't use the contraceptive pill. The Pill is such a no-no for hormonal health that I give it a separate chapter ahead.

If you have lost your estrogen to surgery, or if you are menopausal or past menopause, or if you are a male with low estrogen, then *do* investigate using estrogen. It will help you not only to maintain your potency and your brain, but, as we will see, it will also protect you from cardiovascular disease and immune dysfunction. Like the Pill, however, there are so many pitfalls to estrogen therapy that I have to give it a chapter of its own.

Dopamine Protector

The third strategy to protect your brain is to maintain dopamine metabolism. Remember, dopamine is the dominant neurotransmitter that controls sexual functions in the sexual areas of the brain. Acetylcholine and dopamine act in concert like twin jets in a rocket engine. And studies in England show that Alzheimer's also involves not only loss of acetylcholine function, but also of dopamine function.[29]

Acetyl-l-carnitine affords some protection to your dopamine[30], but a compound that protects it better is **selegiline hydrochloride** Selegiline used to be freely available in America and Europe before greedy pharmaceutical eyes saw its potential. Now it's a prescription drug in America for treatment of some manifestations of the brain degeneration of usual aging. Most prescriptions, however, are written for normal folk, including numerous celebrities, senators and congressmen in America, who use it as a cognition booster and a preventative of brain aging.

In Europe selegiline is *the* most popular anti-aging substance. Nevertheless, you should know the facts before you choose whether to use it or not. To acquaint you with them, see the chapter ahead, Selegiline For Life.

It will take another 20 years for this new scientific information to penetrate the fusty corridors of medicine.

You can't wait. With usual aging, cognition begins to decline about age 40. Waiting to treat Alzheimer's until the disease becomes manifest, is like waiting for your car engine to seize before you put in any oil. The time to inhibit degeneration of your hormonal systems and your brain is *now*.

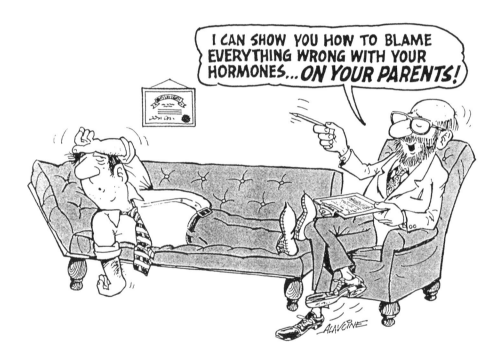

Hormones & Emotions

Marie is a beautiful, vivacious brunette of 28. Rather, she was. Now sitting with hunched shoulders and bloodshot, black-circled eyes, her face is lifeless, set in lines of melancholy. I have seen that mask of female depression many times.

Since her normal pregnancy and easy birth of a healthy son, Marie had sunk into alternating bouts of frenzied activity and deep depression. When six months of multiple antidepressants and psychotherapy failed to fix it, she was sent to me for a last-ditch nutritional supplement program. With a loving husband, and no financial worries, or other definable cause, her physician was at a loss. Privately to me he dismissed the disorder as psychological, "all in her head".

When I told Marie it was completely a physical problem, she sobbed with relief. "I thought I had gone mad," she said. "The psychiatrist diagnosed me as manic-depressive." With the right nutritional and hormonal treatment she was back to happy and beautiful within six weeks.

Studies in America, Canada, France, Italy, Germany, and New Zealand all show that women suffer depression at least twice as frequently as men, and for longer periods. Incidence is even higher during and following pregnancy. After menopause, incidence of female depression rises to astronomical.[1-6] These findings give us all the tools we need to forge the link between your sex hormones and your emotions.

Estrogen Drives Immunity

Let's look first at the dramatic rise in female depression and manic-depression after normal births.[7] Fortunately, most women suffer no more than postpartum "blues". Depressive symptoms peak about a week after birth then gradually disappear.[8] But for one in every nine births, symptoms progress into major depression, typified by self neglect and poor child care, increased use of alcohol and drugs, and increased risk of suicide.[9] Episodes can begin anytime up to three months after childbirth, and continue for up to two years.[10,11]

The clue to why women suffer this problem comes from new research on the female immune system. In order to successfully grow the fetus, and then nurture the helpless infant, without disease claiming her or her baby, the woman's immune system has to be much stronger than the male's.[12]

The key to female immune strength is estrogen, or rather estrogens, because there are many of them.   Estrogens represent   the   latest   hormone   development   on   the evolutionary ladder. All your sex hormones are made in a sequence of chemical steps from **cholesterol**, yes cholesterol, the supposedly bad for you but in fact vital compound, without which you would quickly die. The estrogens are the final step. Figure 6 shows the main steps of the progression, to illustrate how estrogens are the last (and most complex) development in the sex hormone chain.

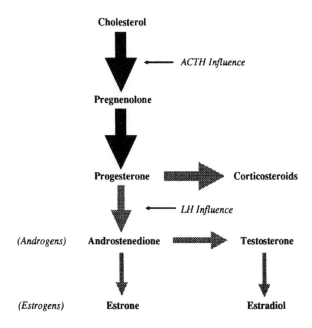

Figure 6. Bodily production of steroid hormones. Size of arrows illustrate progressive reduction in the amount of substrate available.

After puberty the male immune system is more or less set for life. But the female immune system varies enormously every month, and even more during pregnancy. It's all controlled by hormones.

A woman's immunity varies directly with her estrogen. The higher her estrogen levels the stronger her immune response. Prior to ovulation every month, estrogen rises to strengthen immunity, increasing her store of lymphocytes so she can resist bacteria and viruses. The high level of estrogen also affects her brain, revving both acetylcholine and dopamine systems to the point of overactivity in many women. This excess causes the classic symptoms of anxiety, irritability and hypersensitivity of the senses, which constitute the cognitive component of the **premenstrual syndrome (PMS)**.

The high estrogen before ovulation primes the immune system for essential house-cleaning of the uterus and reproductive tract, to protect the descending egg from stray viruses and bacteria, and to clean the womb of debris in preparation for fertilization and implantation.

But at ovulation, estrogen levels drop sharply. Progesterone also increases to further depress immunity. Otherwise the immune system would kill incoming sperm. Even if one sperm did survive, an estrogen-spiked immune system would kill and expel the fertilized egg as a foreign body.

To prevent the immune system killing the fetus, estrogen levels remain suppressed, and progesterone levels remain high, throughout pregnancy. Then, at birth, estrogen levels rebound and progesterone drops dramatically in most women. Immunity rises to its highest level. This miracle of design occurs, so that the mother can resist infection at a critical time of nurture, and can also pass strong immune factors to the immune-weak newborn through her milk.

Estrogen Prevents Depression

The strong estrogen rebound at the birth of her child also stimulates the woman's acetylcholine and dopamine systems of the brain to a frenzy, in some women to the point of madness. This action is offset, however, by a simultaneous rise in the amino acid **tryptophan** which promotes an increase in brain levels of the neurotransmitter **serotonin**. Remember from Chapter 3 how serotonin works to damp down acetylcholine and dopamine activity. That's the way most antidepressants work too, by increasing serotonin activity.

O.K. I hope you're still with me. It's complicated but worth it. In women who get bad postpartum blues, the estrogen rebound is small, and no increase occurs in tryptophan levels. But levels of **cortisol**, the "stress hormone", go through the roof.[7]

In one out of every nine births this hormone imbalance, especially the low estrogen, suppresses the get-up-and-go neurotransmitters in the sexual areas of the brain. Result: major depression, including loss of confidence, confusion, neglect of self and child care, loss of love for the child, continual fatigue, and great unhappiness. Libido is non-existent.

Treatment Strategies

As in the case history of Marie at the start of this chapter, usual medical treatment consists of antidepressants and psychotherapy. Newer drugs such as fluoxetine (Prozac) are often successful at elevating mood to tolerable, because they inhibit the re-uptake of serotonin by nerves, thus increasing its relative brain level, and its tranquilizing effect. But they do nothing for estrogen, dopamine or acetylcholine. So despite the drugs, there's no way out from the fatigue, low self-image, low confidence, impotence, and lack of well-being. You don't see many happy people who have to take antidepressants just to get through their day.

Beyond a bit of handholding, psychotherapy is also unsuccessful.[13,14,15] Psychological techniques are powerless against the postpartum syndrome of depression/impotence, because it is primarily a physical disorder.

Neither the usual drug therapy nor psychotherapy even addresses the real problem - the demon of hormone imbalance. Few physicians have tried it yet, but restoration of normal estrogen levels with exogenous estrogen, and stimulation of acetylcholine with the nutritent **acetyl-l-carnitine** can work wonders.

Because of the absent libido, I suspect that testosterone is also low in women with postpartum depression. No one has yet measured it well.

Remember how dopamine controls testosterone via the hormone cascade from the pituitary. Dopamine levels can be increased easily with a small dose of **selegiline**. This non-toxic strategy may be all that is required to raise testosterone levels.

If the mother has stopped or is stopping breast feeding, then the much stronger drug **bromocriptine** will drop her prolactin like a stone, and can raise testosterone levels within a few days.

These strategies are based only on case histories. They are still speculative because research on female sexual and emotional health is sadly neglected, and controlled trials are non-existent. So don't even think of adopting them on your own. The timing and dosages have to be in concert with your own hormonal cycle. Go see your physician, preferably clutching a sheaf of the medical references given in this chapter. Before you go, you will need a bit more ammunition on testosterone.

Testosterone For Sex and Joy

You know from previous chapters how both males and females require levels of testosterone appropriate to each gender for normal libido. New research shows that adequate testosterone is also essential for normal emotions, especially confidence, friendliness, affection, and joy.

In one study at the University of California, Los Angeles, Dr. Christina Wang monitored the mood and well-being of 54 men with low testosterone levels. Overall the men were irritable, anxious, and angry, and expressed a long list of negative emotions. When they were given sufficient testosterone to raise their levels to normal, every emotion changed in a positive direction.[16] The men became much happier and friendlier.

Endocrinologist Dr. William Brenner at the Seattle Veterans Affairs Medical Center has taken this research one step further. He used drugs to lower testosterone temporarily in healthy men. They quickly became insecure, irritable, and angry, and lost their libidos and zest for life.[17]

We don't know how many women have had their testosterone and emotions damaged by medical drugs, hormonal changes at pregnancy, and gynecological surgery. The medicine men will not measure it for fear of what they will find. If we take libido as a touchstone, it's catastrophic. In American and European clinics, women with low libido constitute about half of all female cases.[18,19]

Outside of clinical cases, a recent study in England examined apparently healthy women aged 35-59. Almost one in every five showed low libido.[20] A similar study in Denmark of 40-year-old women showed that almost *half* of them had low libido.[21]

In 1978 a landmark study of healthy American married couples appeared in the **New England Journal of Medicine**. It showed that over one-third of the wives had lost most or all of their interest in sex and had become sexually dysfunctional.[22] When we compare this finding with the new and extensive, **Sex In America** study, just completed at the University of Chicago, we see a worsening trend over the last 20 years. One-third of all American married women are now frigid. And remember, studies show that low libido and depression form the twin horns of the female hormonal dilemma.[13]

Depression and Menopause

Whoa! say some of my medical colleagues with patronizing smiles. You can't be right that low testosterone is a major cause of female depression. A woman's testosterone level doesn't drop at menopause because the post-menopausal ovaries continue to secrete testosterone. Yet rates of depression go through the roof. So testosterone can't be involved in female depression.

It's time to lay this old bogey to rest. As the medical text-books say, female ovaries do continue to produce testosterone after menopause. But the ovaries are not a woman's main source. Together the adrenals, skin, bodyfat and brain of young women produce far more testosterone than her ovaries. Production by all these sources declines sharply at perimenopause. It's a knock-down, drag-out, big fat lie that female testosterone remains stable. With usual aging, it drops like a brick.

The lie arose from older studies that measured testosterone levels from menopause on. Big mistake. Recent longitudinal studies have measured testosterone levels *before* menopause, during the five years or so of perimenopause. This research shows clearly that testosterone declines in women years before their periods disappear.[23,24]

Especially strong is the research of Dr. Christopher Longcope and colleagues at the University of Massachusetts Medical School. Testosterone levels in healthy women with normal menstrual cycles are about twice as high as in women approaching menopause. By the time women reach menopause, testosterone levels have already dropped to minuscule.

Older studies comparing levels at menopause, then again a year or two later, were looking in the wrong time frame.[25]

It will take years before the new research hits the textbooks, and more than a decade before it becomes public knowledge. By realizing now that female testosterone declines before menopause, you get a jump on the action. Take the research reviewed here to your physician and request that your hormones be restored to young adult levels. If he will not listen, find another physician. The Colgan Institute keeps a list of better informed physicians in America. Phone (619) 632-7722. It could save your mind, your sexuality, your emotions - and your marriage.

To help you further, young, healthy, adult women have the following serum hormone levels:[26,27]

Hormone	Range
Testosterone	30-110 ng/dl
Estradiol*	70-145 ng/l
Progesterone*	0.15-1.5 mcg/l

* Follicular phase of cycle

Note well that the normal female level of testosterone is higher than that of estradiol the primary estrogen. Yet most medicine men ignore the testosterone needs of perimenopausal and postmenopausal women. In fact, most of these women get no hormones at all. Only 20% of postmenopausal women in America are even on estrogen or estrogen/progestins (synthetic derivatives of progesterone).

Trouble is, the out-of-date information in the **Physicians'
Desk Reference**, recommends estrogen only in the case of
vasomotor symptoms such as hot flashes. It repeatedly
states "there is no evidence that estrogens are effective for
nervous symptoms or depression."[27]

No evidence! What sandpile do they have their heads in!
There's a heap of recent studies. In the latest, postmenopausal
women given estrogen showed dramatic improvements in
well-being.[28] If your physician is not up to speed with this
research, find a new one.

Improvement is even better when testosterone is also added.
A good example of the research is the ongoing work of Dr.
Barbara Sherwin, Professor of Psychology at McGill University
in Montreal.[29] She compared women taking estrogen with
those taking estrogen plus testosterone. The women
receiving the added advantage of testosterone, had higher
energy, were more motivated at work, experienced more
positive emotions, and a higher libido. They were also more
frequently sexually aroused, engaged in more sexual
intercourse and had more orgasms. To deprive a women of
testosterone after menopause, or especially after taking
away her ovaries, is female castration.

But, *caveat emptor*. Even those physicians versed in the
use of **Estratest pills** (Solvay Pharmaceuticals), or **Premarin
with testosterone** (Wyeth-Ayerst), which contain methyl
testosterone in addition to estrogen, are working with crude
tools. Also, beware the new rash of anti-aging clinics that
are doing a brisk trade in periodic estrogen/testosterone
injections. As the coming chapters on hormone therapy
show, most hormone replacement strategies are still in the
Stone Age.

Testosterone in Men

Male testosterone levels are not subject to menopause. Nevertheless, many, many men today have low levels. Testosterone deficit is the primary hormonal cause of male impotence.[30] And you have seen already in this chapter how testosterone deficit whacks male emotions.

More evidence to link male sexuality and emotions, comes from the Baltimore Longitudinal Study of Aging. Over many years of measurement, this huge study found that the higher a male's libido, the more likely he is to have positive emotional responses to other areas of his life.[31] In this short book I have room only for these quick examples, but the evidence is now overwhelming that testosterone is the nut of male human life.

If you find love waning, or negative emotions increasing without obvious cause, have your testosterone level checked right away. If it's low, request your physician to restore it pronto to young adult levels. To help you, young, healthy, adult men have the following serum hormone levels:[27]

Hormone	Range
Testosterone	360-990 ng/dl
Estradiol	20-50 ng/l

Remember the average physician knows next to nothing about restoring hormone levels. It's not just a matter of throwing in some exogenous testosterone There are a lot better ways to do it than by using the hormone itself. So before you go, read well the chapters ahead on the **Hormonal Health Program**.

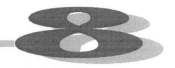

Drugs Hit Hormones

Aging, illicit drugs, illness, pollution, poor nutrition, and couch potatoism can all cause hormonal problems, but the biggest single cause today is - *medication*. The Food and Drug Administration doesn't like you to know that prescription drugs and over-the-counter nostrums cause widespread hormonal damage. If you call them, they deny it. I will tell you the truth. After hundreds of studies, various experts estimate that legitimate drugs, approved by our health authorities, are involved in up to *half* of all cases of hormonal dysfunction.[1]

Medications damn hormonal potency in three main ways: they damage nerves, they damage the vascular system, and they damage the endocrine system. Because many of the drugs attack all three systems, we will save repetition by covering only their main line of attack.

Hormonal Damage

As we have seen, ancient structures in the hypothalamus and striatal cortex control the hormonal components of potency. So we will focus mainly on medications that disrupt these brain mechanisms. Anything that interferes with neurotransmitter function or the hormone cascade, also interferes with every aspect of sexuality. The same drugs that damn libido, arousal, or orgasm, also affect courage, confidence, leadership, intelligence, memory, and passion, even your ability to love.

That's putting it hot and heavy, but the evidence is hot and heavy too. Endocrine problems are widespread and increasing. World experts on sexual dysfunction, Dr. Pierre-Marc Bouloux of the Royal Free Hospital, London, and Professor John Wass of St. Bartholomew's Hospital, London, estimate that up to one-third of all cases of male impotence are caused by endocrine problems.[2] In America alone that totals about 10 million men[3] and unknown millions of women.

I will examine only the most important endocrinopathies. Dr. Roger Kirby, editor of a definitive text on impotence, reports that the most common endocrine symptom is low serum testosterone. Accompanying symptoms are; loss of libido, loss of muscle, loss of strength, increase of abdominal bodyfat, lethargy, fatigue, withdrawal, and depression. If such a syndrome feels familiar, learn this section well. It could save your potency.

Testosterone levels decline with usual aging, such that one American male in every four has insufficient testosterone to remain potent after age 65. The question is: why do they decline?

In women testosterone levels are more variable, and show less decline with usual aging. Nevertheless, world renowned expert Dr. Helen Singer Kaplan puts inadequate testosterone high on the list of female sexual problems.[4]

The biggest single cause of testosterone decline is medication. Drugs that cause sexual endocrinopathies include all those that:

1. Reduce hypothalamus output of gonodotropin releasing hormone.
2. Reduce serum levels of luteinizing hormone.
3. Reduce testosterone production directly.
4. Reduce serum levels of testosterone.

Before discussing each of these categories, I want to mention prolactin again, best known as the milk-stimulating hormone in nursing mothers. As this function might tell you, Nature also designed prolactin to be a strong inhibitor of sexuality.

You saw in Chapter 5 how the hypothalamus normally acts to inhibit prolactin secretion by maintaining specific levels of the neurotransmitter dopamine. If dopamine levels decline, the pituitary produces excess prolactin which destroys both libido and testosterone production.[5,6] It follows that any drug that **decreases** hypothalamic dopamine, or **increases** prolactin production, can cause a decline in hormonal potency.

Anti-hypertensives Cause Impotence

Having added excess prolactin to the potential causes of impotence, let's look at popular prescription drugs that can beat your hormones to a pulp. Most common are the anti-hypertensive agents. Some of them, such as **clonidine**, **reserpine**, and **methyl-dopa** inhibit hypothalamic activity and also elevate serum prolactin levels.

Others, notably the alpha-receptor antagonists, such as **phenoxybenzamine**, reduce production of luteinizing hormone in men. Another category is beta-blockers, such as **propranolol**. The major side effect of beta-blockers is inhibitory action on penile erection. But they also reduce male libido and well-being, so must affect the brain.[7] Although the studies have yet to be done, it's likely that all these drugs can cause similar problems for women.

Vasodilators, such as **hydralazine** can cause both male and female impotence, both by reducing the penile or vaginal blood supply and by inhibiting libido.[1]

A similar attack on libido and blood supply occurs with diuretics, such as **thiazide**, **furosemide**, and **spironolactone**. These diuretics must affect hormone levels also, because they can cause gynecomastia, that is, the growth of female breast tissue in males.[1]

No one has measured it, but women who use diuretics also probably experience an increase in the size of their breasts. It's ironic that breast size, the dominant Western symbol of female sexuality, can be increased by drugs that simultaneously reduce both desire and performance.

Antidepressants Cause Impotence

Almost all antidepressants, including both tricyclics and monoamine oxidase (MAO) inhibitors reduce libido.[1] They have other damaging effects too. The popular tricyclic antidepressant **clomipramine**, for example, causes a variety of potency problems in up to 90% of users, including weakness, fatigue, and confusion.[8]

Other types of antidepressants, such as **fluoxetine** (Prozac), have widespread sexual effects, probably because of their action on the serotonin system in the brain. As usual, controlled measurement of effects on female sexuality is non-existent. But in men, studies on fluoxetine reported in the **Journal of the American Medical Association**, show sexual dysfunction, especially delayed or absent orgasm, in up to 75% of patients.[9]

This side-effect in delaying orgasm is so reliable that fluoxetine is now being paradoxically touted as a *treatment* for sexual dysfunction.[10] For those men who have the problem of premature ejaculation, it may prove helpful. For the majority of us, it's a definite no-no.

In women, fluoxetine is now being prescribed for premenstrual syndrome. Controlled evidence does show some reduction in depression and anxiety in women with severe PMS.[11] But no one bothered to measure how it also kills their sexuality.

We do know that the mental and physical effects of fluoxetine are so bad that more than one-third of subjects withdrew from the study because of side-effects. They would rather suffer their PMS than the debilitating actions of the drug.

Tranquilizers Cause Impotence

Major tranquilizers, such as the popular phenothiazines (e.g. **chlorpromazine**) and butyrophenones (e.g. **haloperidol**) inhibit dopamine action in the brain, and thereby damn sexuality by increasing prolactin secretion.

Minor tranquilizers, such as the benzodiazepines (e.g. **diazepam, chlordiazepoxide**) all have a central depressive effect on the brain that inhibits libido and cognition. Other sedative drugs such as **meprobamate** and the whole class of **barbiturates** have similar depressive effects.[1] Although most of the research is on men, women are likely to be even more sexually inhibited by these drugs, because of their more sensitive testosterone balance.

Thyroid Hormones Cause Impotence

Another endocrine source of impotence is misuse of thyroid medications. The common prescription of thyroid to athletes, and to treat non-specific fatigue, causes many cases of excess levels of thyroid hormone. Excess thyroid in the blood causes increased conversion of testosterone to estrogen.[12] About 70% of males with hyperthyroid conditions show loss of libido, and up to 40% develop gynecomastia.[13] Women are even more likely to lose libido, because their normal levels of testosterone are soon destroyed by excess thyroid.

Conversely, hypothyroidism (low thyroid) also causes impotence. Hypothyroid patients have low levels of testosterone and high levels of the sex killer prolactin.[14]

Anabolic Steroids Cause Impotence

Anabolic steroids including all the testosterones, both prescribed and illegal, can destroy libido in both sexes and erectile function in males. Initially these drugs increase libido. Then, after a few weeks or months, depending on the individual, the form of the drug, and the dose, the high levels of testosterone analogs in the bloodstream signal the hypothalamus to stop production of gonadotropin releasing hormone. This action in turn cuts production of luteinizing hormone and follicle stimulating hormone in the pituitary. Without the steady supply of these hormones, testicular function declines and testosterone production drops to a dribble.

Some anabolic steroids are so effective at producing impotence that they are being tried as male contraceptives. **Nandrolone decanoate** (Deca Durabolin) for example, reduces sperm production to near zero within weeks.[15] So does the **testosterone enanthate** (Delatestryl) form of testosterone.[16]

It's this fall in sperm volume that causes the common shrinking of testicles in male athletes who use anabolic steroids. After a steroid cycle, libido, erection, spermatogenesis, and well-being may take six months or more to recover.[17]

Anabolic steroid users, and patients on cycles of testosterone replacement therapy, often use **human chorionic gonadotropin (HCG)** (Profasi) during and after drug cycles, in attempts to maintain or restore their potency. Theoretically HCG will do the job, but dosage and timing have to be precise.[18] Most physicians have no idea how to do it.

Studies show that the single HCG injection commonly used after a steroid cycle is only marginally effective.[19] But repeated HCG injections, on some arbitrary schedule during or after steroid use, can *worsen* the problem by making the Leydig cells of the testes insensitive to luteinizing hormone. Bingo!   Production of testosterone drops to zero. Bye-bye love, hello tea and slippers.

Oral Contraceptives Cause Impotence

The uncontrolled prescription of oral contraceptives will be remembered in the new millennium, as one of the biggest medical crimes of the 20th century. The Pill has such devastating effects on both health and potency that I give it a separate chapter ahead.

Suffice here to draw from the ongoing research of psychobiologist Dr. Rosemarie Krug, who is a specialist in the effects of contraceptive hormones on sexuality, emotions, and intellectual functions, at the Medical University of Lubeck in Germany. She has found that women on the Pill not only lose much of their sexual desire, but also lose much of their cognitive ability to perceive sexual stimuli and images. Right now 40-50% of all American and European pre-menopausal women are perceiving and thus experiencing their whole lives through the drug-induced fog produced by the Pill. Don't be one of them.

What To Do

The Pill and all the other drugs I have covered, are only the tip of the iceberg of medications that cause impotence. It would fill this whole book to discuss them all. If you are trying to find out about a particular drug, *don't* rely on the **Physicians Desk Reference**. Impotence is conspicuously omitted from lists of side-effects given therein. My best advice is search for studies in the medical reference services on the Internet, or at a university medical library, using the generic name of the medication plus the words "sexual dysfunction".

If you find evidence, take it to your physician and request alternative treatment. There are alternative prescription drugs such as the antidepressants **trazodone** (Desyrel) and **bupropion** (Wellbutrin), the anti-prolactin drug **bromocriptine**, and the anti-hypertensive drugs called **calcium-channel blockers,** which have little effect on hormonal potency. On the contrary, bupropion and some other drugs can *enhance* potency and well-being. Exercise your rights to use them.

It's high time physicians realized that paying with loss of potency for the reduction of symptoms of some other disease, may cause bigger problems than it solves. To help you in your search, common medications that can cause impotence are summarized in the table below.

Common Prescription Drugs
That Can Damage Hormonal Potency

Antihypertensives

Alpha-blockers
 phentolamine (Regitine*)
 phenoxybenzamine
  (Dibenzyline)
 prazosin (Minizide)

Beta-blockers
 propanolol (Inderal)
 metoprolol (Toprol)
 atenolol (Ternormin)

Mixed blockers
 labetalol (Trandate)

Adrenergic blockers
 guanethidine (Esimil)
 guanadrel (Hylorel)
 mecamylamine (Inversine)

Central Sympatholytics
 clonidine (Catapres)
 guanabenz (Wytensin)
 guanfacine (Tenex)
 reserpine (Diupres)
 methyldopa (Aldoclor)

Diuretics
Thiazides
 hydrochlorothiazide (Aldactazide)
 chlorthalidone (Combipres)

Loop diuretics
 furosemide (Lasix)
 bumetanide (Bumex)
 ethacrynic acid (Edecrin)

Potassium-sparing diuretics
 spironolactone (Aldactone)
 amiloride (Midamor)
 triamterene (Dyazide)

Carbonic anhydrose inhibitors
 acetazolamide (Diamox)

Vasodilators
 hydralazine (Ser-Ap-Es)

Note: **Calcium-channel blockers**
are *least* likely to cause hormonal
problems

*Capitalized names in brackets are common American brand names.

Table continued overleaf

Common Prescription Drugs That Can Damage Hormonal Potency (Cont.)

Sedatives
barbiturates
meprobamate (Deprol)

Antidepressants
Trycyclics
amitriptyline (Elavil)
desipramine (Norpramin)
nortriptyline (Pamelor)
doxepin (Adapin)
clomipramine (Anafranil)

MAO inhibitors
phenelzine (Nardil)
isocarboxiazid (Marplan)
tranyleypromine (Pamate)
procarbazine (Matulane)

Anti-asthmatics
ephedrine (Quadrinal)

Cardiac drugs
digoxin (Lanoxicaps)
disopyramide (Norpace)
verapamil (Calan)
nifedipine (Procardia)

Anticholinergics
diphenhydramine (Benadryl)
atropine (Donnatal)
propantheline (Pro-Banthine)
benztropine (Cogentin)

Major Tranquilizers
Butyrophenones
haloperidol (Haldol)

Phenothiazines
chlorpromazine (Thorazine)
mesoridazine (Serentil)

Thioxanthenes
chlorprothixene (Taractan)
thiothixene (Navane)

Anxiolytics
Benzodiazepines
diazepam (Valium)
chorazepote
chlordiazepoxide (Librium)
triazolam (Halcion)

Anti-androgens
cimetidine (Tagamet)
ketoconazole (Nizoral)

*Capitalized names in brackets are common American brand names.

Table continued overleaf

Common Prescription Drugs That Can Damage Hormonal Potency (Cont.)

Hormone analogs
  stanozolol (Winstrol)
  oxymetholone (Anadrol)
  fluoxymesterone (Halotestin)
  gonadotropin releasing
    hormone
  histrelin (Supprelin)
  nafarelin (Synarel)
  nandrolene decanoate
  testosterone enanthate
  human chorionic
    gonadotropin (HCG)

Oral Contraceptives
  norethindrone and estradiol
    (Brevicon)
  ethynodiol and estradiol
    (Demulen)
  norethindrone and mestranol
    (Norinyl)
  norgestrinate and estradiol
    (Ortho-cyclen)
  levonorgestrel and estradiol
    (Triphasil)

*Capitalized names in brackets are common American brand names.

*Sources: Physician's Desk Reference 1995, Colgan Institute, San Diego, C.A. Kirby RS, ed., **Impotence**, Oxford: Butterworth-Heinnemann, 1991.

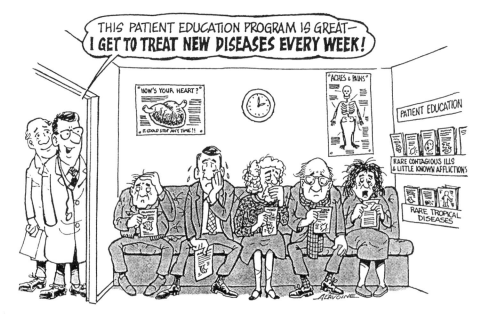

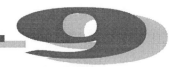

That Pesky Pill

Use of female sex hormones exploded in the early '60s, when GD Searle rolled out the first American oral contraceptive - **Enovid**. This little estrogen bomb created a booming new market, seething with drug companies desperate for plunder. In the stampede to fatten the bottom line, women's health was trampled underfoot.

Profits from early versions of the Pill were equaled only by the widespread disease it caused. In 1969, medical journalist Barbara Seaman wrote a blistering expose'. Her book, **The Doctors' Case Against The Pill,** was also a revelation of hidden medical crimes of the American health care system.[1]

At that time medicine still enjoyed the same holiness and immunity from public criticism as religion. Attacking it as she did, roused powerful forces of revenge. Seaman was fired from her job and reviled by corrupt medical interests of the day. Meanwhile, activists shouting her slogan nationwide,

"Love with the Pill can cripple and kill."

prompted government hearings under Senator Gayelord Nelson that quickly revealed the truth of Seaman's analysis.

But it was already too late. It would take this whole book to document the huge variety of diseases promoted by early versions of the Pill, so I have space only to focus on one example - cancer. During the early '70s, rates of endometrial cancer went through the roof, closely followed by breast cancer. Studies showed that estrogen drugs increased the risk of endometrial cancer by 1400%.[2]

Bloated with money from these drugs, pharmaceutical companies hired medical front men to bamboozle the FDA and the medically unsophisticated press of that time. Then they quickly and quietly lowered the estrogen doses. They also added **progestins** (man-made analogs of progesterone). Endometrial cancer rates declined.[2] Such was the sanctity of medicine that, apart from a few small settlements, this massive medical blunder was swept under the rug.

Today, the public have realized that most medicine is simply trade for profit, no holier than making widgets or flipping burgers. When widgets kill people or burgers poison them, the tradesmen have to take the consequences. If the estrogen disaster was repeated today, the ensuing class-action suits would make the $4.5 billion settlement against breast implants look like parking change.

Excess Estrogen

Why am I so bitter about the early estrogen pills? Because at that time, scientists were already well aware of the dangers of excess estrogen. Women with high estrogen levels were known to have higher risks of reproductive cancers. Science established over half a century ago that breasts of high-estrogen women tend towards ample, because estrogen signals tissue growth in the body, especially in the reproductive system. Excess estrogen leads to tissue overgrowth. Women in America, for example, have much higher estrogen levels than women in Japan, and larger breasts, and for many decades have had four to six times the Japanese rates of breast cancer.[3]

Errant drug companies quickly added progestins (progesterone mimics) to their early high-estrogen contraceptive, because it was well known that progesterone selectively suppresses estrogen action. In the uterus, progesterone signals growth cessation and sloughing off of cells. No surprise then that endometrial cancer rates rose astronomically with high-dose estrogen alone, and fell just as quickly with low-dose estrogen plus progestins. The medical name for it today - **opposed estrogen** - speaks volumes.

Out, Out Damned Progestins

Why wasn't progesterone added to estrogen pills in the first place? And why were synthetic progestins added instead of natural progesterone? Thereby hangs another tale of medical misdemeanor.

One reason progesterone wasn't part of the mix from the beginning, was that it counteracts estrogen, and therefore could make the pill ineffective. This notion has since proved false.

A second reason is the almighty dollar. There's no money in progesterone, because patent laws forbid any drug company exclusive rights to it. So their boffins busied away inventing progestins, man-made molecules similar to progesterone, but profitably patentable.

Trouble is, progestins don't have the same chemical or emotional effects as progesterone. Natural progesterone tends to have sedative and calming effects on brain function.[4] It is used with some success in treatment of premenstrual syndrome.[5] In contrast, science has known since the 1960s, that many man-made progestins generate negative emotions, including the very anxiety/depression roller-coaster of PMS that progesterone alleviates.[6,7]

So progestins were not expected to sell well. When estrogen-induced disease finally forced their use, many women felt so bad on them, they stopped using hormones entirely. If you are on opposed estrogen therapy and find yourself screaming at your children or your spouse, or depressed or confused for no good reason, ask your physician about switching to natural progesterone as the estrogen control agent. Insist on it.

Estrogen Causes Breast Cancer

Medical scientists have known since animal studies in the '50s that estrogen causes breast cancer. But such is the power of commerce, that pharmaceutical companies convinced the U.S. Food and Drug Administration that tissue overgrowth caused by estrogen in human breasts was essentially harmless. Bull pucky! There is a mountain of evidence that one common form of overgrowth, **ductal hyperplasia** (breast lumps) produces precancerous lesions.[8] The latest issue of the **Johns Hopkins Medical Letter** warns women who have breast lumps against estrogen therapy.[9]

"Not to worry" said the pharmaceutical pundits, "Addition of progestins will fix it anyway." Bull pucky again! Scientists have known for decades that progesterone suppression of estrogen is highly selective. Though it readily controls pathological growth in the uterus, it has only a small protective influence on the breast.

The huge Nurses Study trial by researchers at Harvard Medical School followed 70,000 postmenopausal nurses for 10 years. Results have just confirmed again what we knew 30 years ago. After five years of therapy with either estrogen alone, or estrogen plus progestins, risk of breast cancer increased by 32%.[10] The progestins gave no protection at all. A good chunk of the increase in breast cancer in postmenopausal women in America, has estrogen therapy as its root cause.

Young women are also caught in estrogen's breast cancer trap. A pile of studies shows without doubt, that the estrogen in oral contraceptives, has caused a major chunk of the increase in breast cancer in young women, not only in America, but all over Western Society.[11] Indeed one of the questions now used to predict the risk of breast cancer in young women who go to their doctor because they develop breast lumps or tenderness is, "How early did you begin using the Pill?"[12]

In the latest study, Dr. Louise Brinton and colleagues of the U.S. National Cancer Institute in Bethesda, Maryland, compared 2,200 breast cancer patients with 2,000 healthy women in Atlanta, Seattle, central New Jersey and Puget Sound. Women under 35 who had used the Pill for as little as 6 months, *almost doubled* their risk of breast cancer. Those who started the Pill before age 18, and had taken it for 10 years or more, *tripled* their risk.

It's no surprise then that the incidence of breast cancer has surged in recent decades. Incidence has been rising ever since estrogen pills were first introduced in the '60s.

Worse, so has the breast cancer death rate,[13] indicating that this cancer is now more virulent than it was 30 years ago. I show in my book **Prevent Cancer Now,** how medicine is curing a smaller percentage of breast cancer cases than it did in 1965.[14] Estrogen use is a major suspect in the increased deadliness of this disease.

Though incorrect estrogen therapy is not the only cause of our epidemic of breast cancer, it is one documented risk we can eliminate. And we should, pronto. Breast cancer is now the leading cause of cancer death in women in America, Canada, Britain, most of Europe, Australia and New Zealand.[13]

America, which has the highest use of estrogen replacement therapy, has the highest rate of breast cancer among postmenopausal women. New Zealand, which has the most liberal attitudes towards prescription of the Pill to young women, has the highest rates of all.[13]

Don't fret. If you give up the Pill, risk of breast cancer drops to baseline in two years.[10] And, if you "just have to" use the Pill to prevent pregnancy, as so many women tell me, the coming chapters on hormone therapy show how you can cut your risk to a minimum.

The Pill Kills Sex

Another nasty little secret that drug companies don't want women to know about the Pill is - it knocks your sexuality flat. And, along with it goes much of your well-being, energy, confidence, and zest for life.

Knowing this from the getgo, medicine men have done a great public relations job to convince women of the opposite. It is true that the Pill does relieve the anxiety of unwanted pregnancy that otherwise inhibits sexual intercourse. But, in many women, the increase in peace of mind is more than offset by the loss of sexual emotions that pervade every facet of their lives.

It doesn't usually happen overnight. Destruction of female sexuality by current versions of Pill can take years. Just like development of breast cancer from the same source, it's insidious and symptomless, so subtle that most victims don't notice until it emerges full-blown. When they finally present with complaints of lost libido, depression, and fatigue, all the usual tests show nothing. The typical medical response is, "Well, you're over 30. You should expect some reduction of the flush of youth."

Evidence of lost libido caused by the Pill, began to surface along with evidence of cancer, about a decade after it went on the market. With the high estrogen levels of the early Pill, some women went asexual within weeks of starting it.[15] And studies in the '70s showed that the majority of women using the early Pills quickly lost their sexuality.[16]

The Pill Whacks Testosterone

We now know one way that the Pill kills sexuality. As I reviewed in Chapter 4, testosterone drives both male and female libidos. Recent evidence shows that the Pill progressively lowers female testosterone levels.[17] As testosterone also acts as an estrogen control agent, this effect also helps explain the Pill's action in promoting a wide range of diseases.

Drug companies realized that their profits would disappear quicker 'n a bug in a blender, if the Pill became branded as a disease-causing sex killer. So they promoted research on satisfied Pill users, and once more gulled a naive press into extolling its virtues.

But sex researchers were not so easy to gull. Prominent among them are Dr. Barbara Sherwin of McGill University in Montreal and Dr. J. Bancroft of Edinborough University in Scotland. They showed that women with normal sexuality, gave up the Pill when they felt its negative effects on their emotions and sex life.[18] In a follow-up study they also showed that women who continue to use the Pill have lower hormonal potency than non-users, and are satisfied with minimal sexual relationships, or none at all.[18]

Other researchers followed women who had just started on the Pill, and compared them with women being fitted with intrauterine devices (IUDs) at about the same time. Over the following year, the sexuality of the IUD users increased. The libido and sexuality of the Pill users progressively declined. In some subjects sexuality disappeared altogether, and was replaced by negative emotions and depression.[19]

"Be fair" said one of my medical colleagues, "They have changed the Pill based on this research." Indeed they have. Now there are all sorts of cunning hormone brews, monophasic, diphasic and triphasic, with a multitude of forms of estrogen and progestins. To be fair, I will look at the latest research on one of the best, **Synphasic** made by Syntex Laboratories in Canada.

This pill has a low dose of **ethinyl estradiol,** 35 micrograms per day, for Days 1-21 of the menstrual cycle, plus the progestin **norethindrone** 500 micrograms for Days 1-7, 1000 micrograms for Days 8-16 and 500 micrograms for Days 17-21. Days 22-28 are pill-free. A clever little mixture that is reliably contraceptive, Synphasic also has other effects that are not so endearing.

The Pill Whacks Emotions

Dr. Barbara Sherwin and colleagues gave Synphasic to healthy women as a treatment for mild to moderate premenstrual symptoms, but they were really interested in effects on sexuality. So they measured libido and emotional aspects of potency in these women, and compared them with a control group given placebo pills.

By the third month, the sexual potency of the control group remained unchanged. The Pill group however showed a huge loss of libido throughout their cycles. The Pill did reduce some premenstrual symptoms of depression, but only by what the researchers called a "leveling off" of positive emotions too.[20] It reduced the women's capacity for sorrow only by also reducing their capacity for joy.

This loss of emotional potency brings to mind the lines of poet and philosopher Kahlil Gibran, when he is discussing the abandonment of love:

> Where you shall laugh
> But not all of your laughter
> And you shall weep
> But not all of your tears.[21]

I suspect that the sexual and emotional prison created by the Pill, becomes permanent for many women who use it for a long time. They don't feel great sadness, but they no longer feel great passion either. They have lost their zest.

Why else have so many women lost their sensuality? The latest and most careful sexual survey ever, **Sex In America**, shows that one-third of American women have entirely lost their interest in sex.[22] That's devastating when you know that the same research also shows that general happiness in life is strongly linked with an active sex life.

Research by Dr. Mary Harward at the University of Florida, Gainsville, and Dr. Jack Ende at Boston University, indicates an even worse situation. They have found that more than half of all women patients presenting to general medical practice have some form of sexual dysfunction.[23]

Are women simply less sensual than men to begin with? No way! A comprehensive 14-year survey of young American college women shows that 90% have very active sex lives.[24]

Does female sexuality fade after age 25 or so, when college life is past? No way again! The evidence shows just the opposite. Healthy female sexual potency increases from the early 20s into the late 30s.[25] What seems to have happened in Western Society, where 40-50% of women use the Pill, is ***chemical castration.***

One young woman that the Colgan Institute saved from this fate aptly described life on the Pill:

> I'd forgotten what real passion or real sex felt like. Life was sooo.... so-so, hum-a drum drum.

Don't allow yourself to become one of the victims.

It's likely that the widespread disease, and the sexual and emotional damage caused by the Pill, is also accompanied by intellectual damage. I hope that effective women's activists such as Fran Visco and Kay Dickerson of the Women's Breast Cancer Coalition, push to make research on these problems a national priority. It's far more important to protect women's hormonal health, than to waste endless time and money on "Ms", "fireperson", "unisex", and all the other language-mangling, gender-neutering fop of political correctness.

When they come of age, I will be quick to advise my daughters never to use the Pill. Many intelligent young women are already getting the message. In successive surveys of the sexual habits of American college women over 14 years, the percentage with active sex lives remained stable at about 90%. The percentage using oral contraceptives, however, fell by 20%.[24] Smart.

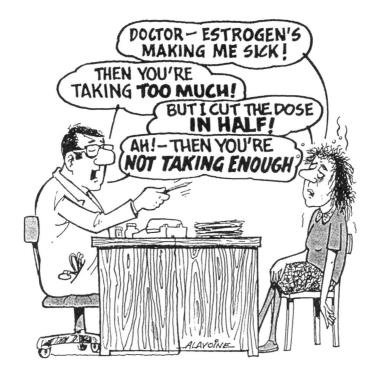

10

Prostate Problems

You may have no prostate problems - yet. But, unless you take the right precautions, you very likely will. The American Prostate Society reports that four men in every five develop prostate overgrowth. And up to 90% of men suffer one of the three forms of prostatitis (inflamatory disease of the prostate).[1] So even if your prostate is clean as a whistle - read on.

The male prostate is a doughnut-shaped gland surrounding the urethra (urine canal) just where it leaves the bladder. Whenever you ejaculate, it releases milky, alkaline, seminal fluid that mixes with sperm and helps protect them from acidity. In young men the prostate isn't a problem. But, about age 30, sometimes earlier, males start converting more of their testosterone into another form called **dihydrotestosterone**. That's the troublemaker.

In combination with some other compounds, increased dihydrotestosterone causes male pattern baldness. It also causes your prostate to grow.[2,3] This overgrowth, called **benign prostatic hypertrophy**, eventually leads to prostate cancer in most men. But they never know. The prostate cancer remains localized lifelong, without symptoms. The majority of men with prostate cancer die from other causes.[4]

Prostate Surgery

Nevertheless, between 1980 and 1990, incidence of known prostate cancer in America increased by 50%.[5] This increase partly results from increasing use of the **prostatic specific antigen (PSA)**, and the **transrectal ultrasound** tests, which can diagnose even microscopic cancers that previously went unnoticed.[6]

Mainly as a result of these tests, surgery of the prostate, sometimes done on mere suspicion of cancer, or even for prostatitis or benign prostatic hypertrophy, has grown to monstrous proportions. From 1984 to 1990, radical prostatectomy operations (removal of the prostate) in America jumped by 600%[7]. And fees rose to $37,000 a pop.[4]

Fine and dandy if these medical machinations increased the number of cancer cures. But US National Cancer Institute figures show just the opposite. The death rate from prostate cancer has risen steadily in America since 1960.[5] Far from improving survival, all this surgery seems to be hastening patient demise. The latest study in the **Journal of the American Medical Association** shows that, on average, radical prostatectomy fails to prolong life by even *one month*, over no treatment at all.[6]

Why am I putting these cancer horrors in a book on hormonal health? Because, if this surgery doesn't kill you, it will likely render you impotent, or make sex so painful you avoid it ever more.[6] Yet health "care" literature has Americans so scared of prostate cancer, the PSA and other tests have become a fixture of annual physicals. And at the first hint of trouble, men are led to surgery like lambs to slaughter.

In a case just published by the American Medical Association, perhaps to stem this tide of unnecessary surgery, a 72-year old sexually potent man was diagnosed with minute localized prostate cancer. On the best predictor of prostate cancer spread, the **Gleason Score**, he had a low risk that the cancer would mestatisize before he died in his 80s of other causes. Yet his oncologist, urologist, and radiotherapist all recommended immediate action.[8] This guy was in luck, however. He was also counseled by Dr. Peter Albertson, head of urology at the University of Connecticut. Albertson correctly advised "watchful waiting".

Incidentally, external beam radiation therapy and hormone therapy, the other two main treatments, have an even worse outcome than surgery. More than 50% of all radiation patients become impotent.[9] With hormone therapy impotence is virtually certain.[10]

Don't become one of these victims. Unless you have distinct prostate symptoms, evidence throughout the world indicates you should avoid the PSA and all the medical palaver that follows a positive test.

This advice may oscillate some medical sphincters, especially in the American Cancer Society so, to put your mind at ease, I better back it up. The US Preventive Services Task Force, the Canadian Task Force on the Periodic Health Examination, and the International Union Against Cancer all recommend *against* routine prostate testing.[2,3,11]   Sweden has the best approach to microscopic or localized prostate cancers - they leave them the hell alone.

Prostate Maintenance

Prevention is an even better idea. I can't tell you what to do, but I can say what I and many of my medical colleagues do.   The usual symptoms of both benign prostatic hypertrophy and prostatitis are reduced urine flow, frequent nocturnal urination, tenderness or pain in the prostate, and pain or burning during urination or during or after intercourse. At the first sign, which may occur at age 40 or even before, we tackle it like this.

First, cut down on animal protein which may be pushing your dihydrotestosterone too high. Second, cut all animal fat. Third, cut polyunsaturated fats. In my book, **The New Nutrition**, I review the evidence showing that most polyunsaturated fats are just as bad as animal fat.[12] Fourth, cut down on coffee, spicy and high-acid foods, and alcohol, especially red wine and strong liquor, all of which aggravate prostatitis.[1]

Fifth, supplement with a tablespoon of organic flax oil, the only vegetable oil that has the right combination of omega-3 and omega-6 essential fatty acids.[11]   Keep it refrigerated. Remember, all good food is food that goes bad quickly, including the good oil.

Sixth, empty the prostate of seminal fluid at least once a week by sexual intercourse or, if necessary, by masturbation. Studies indicate that prostate fluid may become stagnant and provide a breeding ground for any of the 200 known bacteria that can cause prostatitis.[1]

Seventh, ensure that your daily vitamin/mineral supplements contain zinc picolinate, pyridoxine, and silica. All three nutrients help to prevent prostate overgrowth.

The next step is obvious but, to combat media hype, I have to say it. If you have any prostate symptoms, don't get into testosterone replacement therapy. Even though it may temporarily improve sexuality, exogenous testosterone will worsen prostate problems by providing more of the hormone for conversion to dihydrotestosterone.

Finally, take a daily supplement of the herbs **saw palmetto** and **pygeum**, 200-400 mg per day. These herbs inhibit the enzyme that converts testosterone to dihydrotestosterone, that makes the prostate grow. In Europe, pygeum and saw palmetto have been used successfully for 40 years to inhibit prostatic hypertrophy.[13] In America they are available from the Life Extension Foundation in Florida 1-800-841-5433. By this simple action I and my colleagues intend to take our prostates to the grave untrammeled.

11

Hysterical Surgery

Does it strike you as strange that the two most common major surgeries in the United States are cesarean sections and hysterectomies?[1,2] Every year about 750,000 American women have their babies cut out, and another 700,000 have their uteri cut out.[1-3] Are the reproductive systems of American women so defective they require such frequent butchering?

Curiouser and curiouser. When you look closer at reports of the U.S. National Center for Health Statistics, one in every three American women will have a hysterectomy.[3] Yet, in Britain, only one in every five suffer the same fate.[4] In Norway only one in nine women has a hysterectomy.[5] Are British women grown from sturdier stock than Americans, and are Norwegian women three times as robust?

The worst figures come from California, where *half* of all the women are likely to undergo hysterectomies.[6] Are half the women in California defective, compared with one-third of the rest of American women, compared with one-fifth of British women, compared with one-ninth of Norwegian women? Was Truman Capote correct when he claimed that life in California saps our spunk? I think not!

The Hysterectomy Tragedy

One winter when I was a lad, a local surgeon visited our primary school, because many of the pupils were suffering repeated sore throats. After examining a few of us, he volunteered his time to do mass tonsillectomies on all of us, explaining that it would clear up the problem within a couple of weeks. At that time tonsils were considered useless vestiges of human evolution. So, out they came.

Fortunately I was too sick to participate in the free-for-all, and kept my tonsils intact. My brother, however, was healthy, and lost his pronto. Ever since, he has suffered repeated ear, nose, and throat infections, while I rarely catch anything.

Today, we realize that tonsils form an essential part of the human immune system, to be conserved like gold, except in the direst emergency.

But the female uterus and ovaries, that miraculous complex of reproductive organs that ensures the continuation of humanity, is still considered expendable. I complain many times in this book about medical ignorance. Read on to see how hysterectomy alone justifies every one of my complaints.

Hysterectomy is a pivotal case of medical *male*practice against women because, unlike the recently discovered intricacies of hormonal balance, physicians cannot excuse themselves by lack of knowledge. Fifty-one years ago, on the 29th of October 1945, Dr. Norman Miller, eminent surgeon of the Department of Obstetrics and Gynecology at the University of Michigan, delivered a famous paper to his peers: "Hysterectomy: Therapeutic Necessity or Surgical Racket." First published in the **American Journal of Obstetrics and Gynecology** in 1946, it became a classic, reproduced, quoted and cited in medical journals and popular media worldwide, from that day to this.[7]

Miller stated about the uterus, "Its normal behavior during the non-pregnant state, especially during the menstrual cycle, is one of the more important revelations of our age."(p.804) "Hysterectomy in the absence of pelvic disease cannot be justified any more than can removal of the normal breast or gall bladder."(p.805)

In essence, Miller found that, even in 1945, one-third of the hysterectomies performed in 10 American hospitals showed, "no disease or else disease contraindicating hysterectomy."(p.810) He warned that if these unnecessary hysterectomies continued, "We shall witness a tragedy, painful and far-reaching in its implications."(p.810)

Medical Greedlock

This tragedy is now upon us, even worse than Miller predicted. Recent analyses show that almost *half* of all hysterectomies today are done on healthy uteri and ovaries with no disease whatsoever.[8,9,10]

A representative analysis of 16 years of hysterectomies at the prestigious Mayo Clinic for example, showed that the most frequent reason given for the operation was **pelvic relaxation** (prolapse). As we see in a later chapter, correct hormonal therapy plus correct abdominal exercise can solve many of these cases. In others, corrective surgery can reposition the uterus, thereby saving it and all its vital functions.

The second biggest reason for hysterectomy in the Mayo Clinic study was **sterilization**. Effective, yes. Sterilization by hysterectomy is the exact equivalent of male castration, with all the attendant problems of instant menopause, loss of sexuality, loss of well-being, and increased risk of a host of diseases. Tubal ligation, although it has problems too, is equally effective, a lot safer, and preserves the vital organs.

A third big reason was **menometrorrhagia**. That's medical gobbledegook for excessive irregular bleeding between periods. If a medicine man can't do better than hysterectomy to control such menstrual problems, perhaps he should have become a plumber, where he could work on piping systems that don't have a life of their own.

Together the three diagnoses of pelvic relaxation, sterilization and menometrorrhagia accounted for *three-quarters* of all the hysterectomies. Most of these operations were totally unnecessary.

No doubt the surgeons involved could give you many reasons why they were done. But the rising trend of hysterectomies in Britain reveals the main motivation. Since 1975 most of the rise in British hysterectomies has been in private, fee-for-service hospitals outside the British National Health System.[4] As Mark Twain told us, "Virtue is never as respectable as money."

American medicine has been stuck in this medical greedlock for decades. Between 1988 and 1990, 1,700,000 American women had hysterectomies.[11] The cheapest form is abdominal hysterectomy, at that time about $5,500 a pop.[12] So a conservative estimate of the medical income is *nine billion dollars*. Buys a whole lot of toys.

The Hysterectomy Con

Some physicians I have asked, and some medical reviews, claim that the rise in hysterectomies is demand-based not profit based.[13] That is, more hysterectomies are done today because more women ask for them. This notion sounds new depths of medical fatuity.

If more women are requesting hysterectomies, the immediate question is - Why? The answer is, because doctors have persuaded women and popular media that hysterectomies are innocuous, and will solve multiple physical, emotional, and sexual problems.

Dr. A. Amias for example, consultant gynecologist at prestigious St. George's Hospital in London states:

> Women who have had a total hysterectomy experience the full cycle of sexual response with no impairment of physical satisfaction.[14](p. 609)

To women in sexual pain, such persuasion from high and mighty doctors, is like the voice of God urging them to request a hysterectomy. We will see later just how wrong Dr. Amias is.

Prestigious Mayo Clinic gynecologist Dr. Joseph Pratt says he is approaching the philosophy of "the birthday hysterectomy" for any woman who has pelvic complaints. That is, "let the women have her family, then at her 35th or 36th birthday have a vaginal hysterectomy..."[8] (p.1363) He cites as justification, relief of discomfort, freedom from menses and embarrassing accidents, relief of fear of pregnancy, and even the *cost of tampons*.[8] That makes hysterectomy sound about as harmless as buying the right detergent. Of course women are going to request it.

If purported benefits don't drive enough women to request hysterectomy, then fear might do the trick. Leading gynecologist Dr. Neils Lauersen recommends routine removal of ovaries for all women over 55 who are having hysterectomies, because it eliminates the risk of ovarian cancer which tends to rise with age.[15] Think of the outrage if he suggested the same for men: routine removal of the testicles at age 55, because the risk of testicular cancer rises with age. After you Dr. Lauersen - way after you.

Even though the idea is idiotic, it intimidates a lot of women into compliance. Truth is, ovarian cancer is rare and declining. Only 4% of women get ovarian cancer compared with 32% who get breast cancer.[16] Yet no one in their right mind would suggest routine removal of the breasts to prevent breast cancer.

Lauersen also seems unaware that women who have hysterectomies with ovarian conservation, have a much *lower* risk (less than one quarter of the risk) of developing ovarian cancer than the general female population.[17] Despite the truth, however, pompous pronouncements by almighty doctors can easily scare women into requesting surgery. With sheep-like media stuffed with similar sanctimony, analyses show that rising demand for hysterectomy is all supplier-induced, created by the physicians themselves.[13]

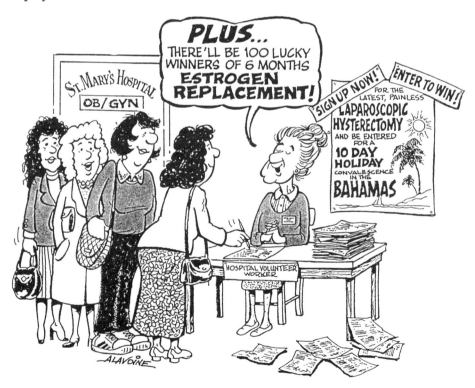

The Miraculous Uterus

Throughout my medical school teaching years, I and many of my colleagues beat our brains out to get it across to students that, unlike man, Nature *never never* designs in discrete units. Every one of her miraculous works does multiple jobs. You have seen in this book for example, how estrogen affects everything from intelligence to emotions to sexuality, even the bloom of your skin and the light that shines in your eyes. It's beyond my comprehension, that presumably intelligent men can act as if the superb architecture of the ovaries and uterus was designed solely to hold the eggs and fetus, and is expendable once that purpose is fulfilled.

Surely these folk do not believe that their puny scalpels, hardly improved on the Neolithic flints of prehistory, can beneficially alter Nature's design with a few crude cuts. They simply do not appreciate the problems of instant and severe menopause that full hysterectomy produces. As you will see ahead, these women get all the menopausal symptoms, triple the risk of heart disease, almost certain osteoporosis, increased risk of colon cancer, increased risk of diabetes, rapid aging of skin, hair, eyes, and mucous membranes, loss of sexuality, loss of memory and intelligence, increased risk of Alzheimer's, and depression in almost half of all cases. If you doubt me, read the medical literature I have cited. Then you will be sure.

I have space for just a few examples of the multiple functions of the uterus, to give you an idea of its complexity. First, your uterus is vital for immunity. Rheumatologist Dr.

Sara Walker at the Veterans Administration Medical Center in Columbia, Missouri, and immunologist Dr. Charles Wira of Dartmouth Medical School, and many other researchers, have compiled a mountain of evidence, that the uterus produces all sorts of **prostaglandins** which regulate the female immune system, even after menopause.[18]

Second, the prostaglandins themselves also have multiple jobs. The uterus produces **prostacyclin**, for example, one function of which is to inhibit the platelets in your blood from clumping into clots. By this action, prostacyclin is directly protective against cardiovascular disease.

Third, despite popular belief among physicians, many women *lose* most of their ovarian function when they lose their uterus, ***despite conservation of the ovaries***.[19] Current research indicates that the uterus may regulate ovarian production via prostaglandins, and by the feedback loop from the cervix to the pituitary gland.[20] Lose your uterus and you've lost much more than the organ itself.

Lost Sex

Sex life after hysterectomy is a lot worse than after menopause. Unlike menopause, where sex and libido show a slow and often manageable decline, hysterectomy stops sexual activity stone dead. This trauma to sexual satisfaction and relationships is all the worse, in that it is frequently suffered by young women whose sexual life prior to surgery may have been abundant.

After the patient has healed, the worst is often yet to come. Hysterectomy almost invariably results in shortening, narrowing, and drying of the vaginal passage, scarring, loss of sensitivity, and frequent pain from scar pressure.[21,22,23] Especially when done for prolapse, one of the most common reasons for hysterectomy, studies show that for up to 50% of patients, the surgery ends sexual intercourse for life.[24]

In addition, no matter how clever the combination of replacement hormones, they cannot compensate for the loss of essential structures of the uterus and cervix. In many women, uterine contractions form part of their sexual arousal and their orgasmic response. In others, the cervix may be essential to trigger orgasm.[21,22] By removing the uterus, sublime sexual relationships are forever ended by the surgeon's knife.

The Ovarian Conservation Scam

Despite the clear synergy of uterine and ovarian functions, hysterectomy is often excused today on the grounds that most modern procedures leave healthy ovaries intact (hysterectomy without oophorectomy). Whoever tells you that is lying through his teeth. Whenever a woman loses her uterus to surgery, her ovaries are damaged beyond repair.

Putting it so heavy raised a lot of hackles among a group of OB/GYN folk, most of whom seemed to think I was questioning their surgical competence. Not at all. Let me spell it out briefly for you, as I did in a much more extended way for them.

Studies show that hysterectomized women who retain their ovaries, develop a much higher risk of cardiovascular disease than women who never have a hysterectomy.[25] They also have a greater risk of depression in later life.[26]   They also lose bone faster[27], making them more prone to osteoporosis, and at an earlier age.   They even develop osteoarthritis more frequently than women who go through menopause intact.[28]

Sexuality also declines.   By retaining some sex hormones, many women who keep their ovaries also retain a near normal libido.   But that does nothing to right the vaginal and other damage of the uterine surgery.   A heap of studies show that despite the desire, sex is often painful or no longer satisfying.[29-31]

Other studies show that hysterectomy with ovarian conservation is often followed by loss of libido.[26,32]   So, despite the supposedly intact ovaries, loss of the uterus still compromises ovarian function, including its production of testosterone and its feedback loop to the brain.   And you have seen earlier in this book, how loss of testosterone function destroys not only libido, but also confidence, well-being, energy, and zest for life.

Many of the women who retain their ovaries after hysterectomy suffer severe menopause when they come of age.   Dr. Anna Oldenhave and colleagues at Leiden University, studied 986 hysterectomized women **who had retained one or both healthy ovaries after hysterectomy**. They found that subjects showed more, and more severe, menopausal symptoms than women who went through natural menopause intact.[33]

The youngest hysterectomized women had the worst problems. Severe hot flashes, night sweats, vaginal dryness, pain, insomnia, and fatigue are hardly conducive to good sexual or emotional relationships. These symptoms also provide a clear indication that, without the uterus, the ovaries cannot produce adequate estrogen, or that if they do, the body can no longer use it properly.

Anyone who snips out the uterus or ovaries willy-nilly, destroys a vital part of your body, your consciousness, your emotional life, and that whole wondrous enigma that you call "myself." Guard these organs well. There's a lot of willy-nilly snipping going on.

Lost Heart

I reviewed the evidence earlier that hysterectomy increases risk of cardiovascular disease by up to 500%, whether or not it is done with ovarian conservation. A young woman given either form of hysterectomy may immediately assume a heart attack risk of 1 in 25, higher than at any time after natural menopause until you reach your 80s.[25]

But that's not the worst loss of heart. For many women given hysterectomies, even partial hysterectomies, the heart goes out of their lives. Passion, love, ecstasy, the emotional essence that drives human achievement, forever after elude them. Up to 50% of these women lapse into repressed anger and depression.[34]

That's why there's no effective outrage against the barbarism of hysterectomy. With less heart for life, and a weaker physical heart to take the strain, hysterectomy reduces untold millions of women to docile tea and slippers. Like the eunuchs of old their spunk is forever silenced.

Avoiding Hysterectomy

The best therapy is to avoid surgery altogether. Be very suspicious of any physician who suggests hysterectomy in the absence of clear disease. Remember, like policemen, physicians are trained in persuasion and intimidation. Unlike policemen, however, they can't detain you. Don't argue. Say no silently and effectively with your feet. Even in cases of clear disease, seek a second and a third opinion.

Be doubly suspicious of gray-haired physicians. I'm serious. Researchers at the University of North Carolina, Department of Medicine compared hysterectomy rates with how long ago the gynecologist went through medical school. Recently trained gynecologists (generally younger and less likely to be graybeards) performed far fewer hysterectomies than those trained 20 years or more ago.[35] So seek a young gynecologist.

Also seek a female gynecologist. For every 100 patients on their respective rosters, males perform 60% more hysterectomies than females. Probably because they have better appreciation of the value of their organs, women are much more likely to recommend alternative treatments.[35]

Finally, contact Hysterectomy Educational Resources and Services (HERS) at 610-667-7757. Started in 1982 by Nora Coffey, herself a victim of hysterectomy, HERS has the most accurate and complete information on the effects of these surgeries. Don't wait until after the operation to have to appeal to HERS for help. Do it now.

12

Who Needs Hormones?

With the solid evidence that estrogen pills cause breast cancer, and that adding progestins or progesterone doesn't stop it, why am I in favor of using hormones? Two reasons. First, it's the amount and timing of the dose that makes the poison. Second, the benefits far outweigh the risks. Once you have a handle on both these factors, you will understand why correct hormone replacement therapy will be one of the greatest advances ever made in human health.

To achieve this advance, our health care system will have to change radically. Even now, as the tarnished tinsel of man-made medicine gives way to the realization that Nature rules, most medicine men still fail to appreciate the complexity of the human body. We are dealing with the balance and orchestration of a system so brilliantly designed, it makes my supercooled, fuel-injected, computer-controlled, 12-cylinder, whiz-bang automobile look like a Tinker Toy.

Know Thy Body

That's the trouble. Medicine still tends to treat the body like one of man's feeble machines. Bung in a bolus of hormones to stop conception by overloading the female hormonal system, like bunging in fuel additives to stop clinker.

Doesn't work. Man-made machines are simple to manipulate, because they are made of discrete units, most of which have no communication with each other. Until you turn them on they are static, dead, unchanging. Their capacity for growth, self-renewal, and response to environmental changes is virtually nil. When in good order, they respond predictably and discretely to simple chemical and electrical inputs - and nothing else.

In contrast, all parts of human bodies are totally integrated, with multiple communication systems linking each part to every other and multiple functions for every part and chemical. A change in any part of the body affects the whole enchilada. I can dent my car's fender on a curb and it carries on regardless. The engine doesn't have any awareness, memory, or response to the dent. But if you stub your toe on a curb, it affects everything, from cognition and emotions, to hormones and immune function, even to the tear glands of your eyes and the sounds coming out of your mouth.

Unlike machines, bodies are also alive, responding 24 hours a day, every day, in infinitely variable ways, to every chemical, electrical, magnetic, and tactual input from the air, food, water, and environment, even the pull of the moon and the change of the seasons.

Bodies also have an internal, genetically driven program of growth and change, so complex that science is only nibbling at the edges of understanding. Whenever you put a drug or anything else into your body, its response is the reaction to that input, *plus* its own internal program, *plus* the sum of all other inputs it is also responding to at that time.

When I was a visiting researcher at Rockefeller University in New York, for two years I had the privilege of working with many great scientists. Three Nobel laureates had labs within strolling distance, and I could knock on their doors and impose myself for lunch any day of the week. Of all that I learned from them, most important was their great humility when faced with the complexity of living flesh.

Once you appreciate the miracle of the human body, it's obvious how incorrect hormone therapy causes disease. If you give estrogen to young women with a program of abundant internal estrogen already, then you should expect the excess to cause mischief, especially wild tissue growth in the breasts and reproductive system.

Studies of young British women, show exactly how the dose makes the excess that makes the poison. Breast cancer risk is directly related to estrogen dose. Risk rises sharply when the Pill contains more than 50 micrograms of estrogen a day.[1] That's only 50 one-thousandths of a milligram, much *less* than in many current forms of Pill. For most young women, the excess of estrogen required to stop conception is clearly poisonous.

Pharmaceutical companies have known all this for years and are racing to get out of the estrogen contraception market before they are legally forced out. New contraceptives such as the B-Oval pill use no estrogen at all. They should be hitting the market a few months after publication of this book.

Menopausal Hormone Replacement - Yes!

Menopause is an entirely different story. When the program of internal estrogen manufacture has declined by loss of ovarian function, then moderate estrogen pills are unlikely to push bodily estrogen into excess. Because estrogen is required for everything from brain function and emotions, to maintenance of the skin, hair, and mucous membranes, estrogen replacement provides many benefits at this stage of your life.

"Wait a minute," say the critics. "Menopause is a natural event. Why should we interfere with the natural drop in estrogen levels." This naive view may have had some credence in Victorian times, when most women died before age 50. But during this century, average female lifespan in some Western countries has increased to over 80. Women now live as much as half their lives after menopause.

For those given surgical menopause, it's a lot longer than that. One-third of American women now enter menopausal age without their ovaries.[2] Unless given continuous hormone replacement, they are faced with 50 years of disability and degeneration.

Female Catastrophe

A decade ago my indictment of menopause as the cause of many diseases was thought extreme. I was accused of everything from misogyny to a criminal conspiracy against women. With the mountain of evidence since then, smart women and their physicians are finally coming around. Leading the parade is New York gynecologist Robert Wilson. Author of the bestseller **Feminine Forever**, he calls menopause the "staggering catastrophe" of women's health, that leads to "fast and painful aging."[3]

So far medicine has done little to tackle this catastrophe, beyond minimal palliative treatment of menopausal symptoms, and crude hormone replacement for a minority of women. Unfortunately, in America, strident feminists of the '70s and '80s bear a lot of the blame for this lack of effective health care. Such was their bitter rhetoric against anyone who dared cast menopause as a female deficiency, that many leading scientists, who had no other motive than to advance human health, withdrew from this area of research.

Even now, reportedly responsible organizations, such as the National Woman's Health Network, sprinkle their otherwise admirable emphasis on nutrition and exercise, with such invective against physicians and pharmaceutical companies, that few will risk the hassle of women's health research.[4] Egged on by rapacious (and mostly male) lawyers, they stand ready with "boiler plate" class action suits, to threaten indiscriminately both good and bad developments in female medicine.[5]

But times they are a-changing. Sufficiently so for me to write this book. Informed women now realize that the "natural" event of menopause causes degenerative processes of aging, in exactly the same way that the "natural" drying and stiffening of joints causes osteoarthritis. With our already long lifespan likely to extend even further, smart folk understand that menopause creates a long-term hormone deficiency disorder.

It's high time. As we will see, by focusing on short-term palliative treatment of menopausal symptoms, health care up to the 1990s has created the epidemics of female osteoporosis, cardiovascular disease, colon cancer, and Alzheimer's, now rampant throughout Western society. The good news is that correct hormone replacement can prevent the major part of all these dire diseases.

Perimenopause

Before you adopt a prevention program, you have to know when to begin. The correct time is at **perimenopause**, the five years or so before menopause. Most physicians still seem to know little or nothing about it. In June 1995, endocrinologist Dr. Howard Zacur of Johns Hopkins Hospital in Baltimore said it right, "Doctors were simply unaware of the existence of perimenopause."[3]

A new Gallup Poll shows that the majority of American women are not happy at all with their doctor's knowledge or treatment of menopause.[3] So the medicine men have a lot of learning to do - and you have to tell them.

With usual aging, perimenopause begins between ages 40-45. Estrogen, progesterone, and testosterone levels lose their rhythmic cycles and begin to decline. Energy drops, and sexuality wanes. For many women libido disappears entirely. Headaches begin. Periods become irregular. Minds become foggy, confused, forgetful. Skin and mucous membranes start to dry, thin, and wrinkle. Hair starts to turn grey, sparse, and brittle. Eyes fade. Emotions swing towards anxiety and irritability. Incidence of clinical depression rises astronomically.[6,7]

Eight out of every 10 women in Britain and America suffer some degree of perimenopause, lasting up to five years. And many of them have been misdiagnosed as having everything from schizophrenia to cancer. If you fit any of the symptoms, then read Dr. Lila Nachtigall's excellent book, **Estrogen: The Facts Can Change Your Life**.[8] Take it to your physician.

Perimenopause is the perfect time to begin *judicious* estrogen/progesterone/testosterone therapy, because then the exogenous hormones do not create an excess, but are simply replacing a failing internal supply.

Even the studies of contraceptive pill use and breast cancer that I reviewed in Chapter 9, confirm this change from excess to replacement, as the female internal life program proceeds. When you examine different age groups within these studies, you see that cancer risk *declines* sharply at age 40-45. That's in contrast to most cancer risks, which *increase* with age. The best explanation is that the estrogen contraceptives are no longer overloading and poisoning the system, but simply bringing levels back up to normal.

The benefits of hormone replacement therapy at perimenopause and thereafter, outweigh by far any small risk that remains. Previous chapters have shown you how estrogen and testosterone maintain your sexuality, and protect your memory, intelligence and emotions. If that's not enough to convince you, read on to discover how estrogen also protects you against a mountain of aging and degenerative disease. And eliminating the small increase in the risk of breast cancer caused by taking estrogen, is a piece of cake.

13

Hormone Benefits

Cardiovascular disease kills 53% of all American women over 50.[1] To put that figure in perspective, breast cancer kills only 4%. To put it more in perspective, figures from the U.S. National Center for Health Statistics, and from the American Heart Association, show that, cardiovascular disease now kills more American women than men.[1]

The female pattern of death, however, is different from that of males. Until menopause, women have a much lower risk of all cardiovascular diseases. Then, over the 15 years after menopause, risk rises rapidly, even surpassing male risk for some heart problems. Deaths from coronary heart disease total only 2 per 100,000 women aged 30-34, about a quarter of the male death rate. But by ages 55-59, the female death rate jumps to a massive 106 per 100,000.[2] A heap of studies from endocrinology to epidemiology, show that loss of estrogen via menopause is the major cause.[3,4]

Estrogen Saves Hearts

Up to this decade, scientists had little idea how estrogen protects your heart. Now evidence is pouring in from every direction. Research by Dr. William Schnaper, Associate Professor of Pediatrics at Northwestern University, shows that estrogen enhances the growth of new blood vessels. Research by Dr. Mark Nelson at Vermont College of Medicine, shows that estrogen causes blood vessels to relax and increase blood flow. Research by Dr. Geoffrey Toffler and colleagues at Harvard Medical School, shows that estrogen increases one clot-dissolving factor in the blood and also reduces the blood-clotting factor, **fibrinogen**.[1,5] It's a v-e-e-e-e-ry busy hormone.

Best established is the research that estrogen improves cholesterol levels. The Postmenopausal Estrogen/Progestin Intervention Trial (PEPI), followed 875 women for three years. Results published in 1995, show that estrogen, or estrogen plus progestins, raises high-density liproproteins (HDL) (the 'good' cholesterol), and lowers low-density lipoproteins (LDL) (the 'bad' cholesterol). Most important for your consideration of hormone replacement therapy, those women who were taking estrogen plus *natural progesterone* showed the biggest improvements.[6,7]

How much does estrogen reduce your risk of heart disease? A helluva lot! Eleven published studies show that cardiovascular risk is reduced in estrogen users by more than *half*.[8] So, if anyone tells you that postmenopausal estrogen therapy is unnecessary for optimal health - don't believe them.

Estrogen For Bones

Osteoporosis, the weak bones disease, used to be uncommon. Today it afflicts one in every two American women over 50 years of age. **The Harvard Medical School Newsletter** calls it, "the silent epidemic."[9]

Silent yes, but not invisible. In my lectures on hormones, I used to show slides of mothers, similar in height to their adult daughters, who, after menopause, shrank in stature by as much as 13 inches.

I say "used to show," because one of my medical colleagues recently sent me worse slides of women with osteoporosis. They had lost so much bone in the spine, it could no longer support the weight of their heads and arms. They were permanently bent double. Their rib cages pressed continually on their pelvic bones, putting them in constant agony.

After one showing to a public audience, I realized it was too depressing for women, to see such examples of the disease with which they currently have a 50/50 chance of ending their lives.

My own reaction is not depression but anger. Yours should be anger too. The 25,000,000 cases of osteoporosis in America alone,[10] are a monstrous indictment of our health care system, because it is an almost completely preventable disease.

I cover all the details and the evidence for the nutritional and exercise steps necessary to prevent osteoporosis in my book, **The New Nutrition**.[11] An outline of the program from that book is given in the table below. Over the past decade, we have used it successfully with hundreds of cases of women with bone loss, referred by their physicians to the Colgan Institute for nutritional help, because they have shown only marginal improvements on estrogen therapy alone. Combined with estrogen, and natural progesterone, this program not only prevents further bone loss, but reliably re-builds bone strength.

Save 'Dem Bones Program
1. Avoid very high protein diets.
2. Avoid meal replacement drinks containing casein, lactalbumin, egg white.
3. Avoid salt.
4. Alcohol. Drink only beer or wine and a maximum of 2 glasses daily.
5. Coffee. Drink a maximum of 2 cups daily.
6. Use a high potency multi-mineral supplement daily containing at least 500 mg calcium, 500 mg magnesium plus all essential trace minerals.
7. Use a high potency, complete, multi-vitamin supplement daily.
8. Eat a low-acid diet of 25-30% protein, 45-55% carbohydrates and 15-20% fats.
9. Do weight-bearing exercise (see chapter ahead).
10. Use a modicum of estrogen (see chapter ahead).
11. Use a modicum of progesterone (see chapter ahead).
12. Follow the **Hormonal Health Program**.

Source: Colgan M. The New Nutrition, Reference 11.

Some women's groups advocate the use of similar nutrition and exercise programs, but without estrogen or estrogen/progesterone. To do so shows crass ignorance of the medical literature. The function of estrogen in maintaining bone was established over 50 years ago by Dr. Fuller Albright, who first showed that postmenopausal women shed bone faster than last year's fashions.[12]

Way back then some physicians objected, saying that Albright was only measuring the natural effects of aging on bone, not the effects of estrogen. This silly myth still persists today among some activist groups, despite a mountain of evidence to the contrary. Their strident nonsense has condemned many thousands of women to decades of unnecessary suffering.

Start Protecting Your Bones Now

To cover all the evidence that estrogen is essential for bone would take this whole book. Pertinent examples will have to suffice. Dr. Robert Lindsay of Columbia University and his colleagues, for example, first showed 20 years ago, that young women who have their ovaries removed, and thus lose most of their estrogen, start to lose bone right away. Only three years after the surgery, they have much weaker bones than women who have the forms of hysterectomy that leave their ovaries intact.[13]

Other studies show that the amount of bone loss depends not on age, but on the time that has passed since loss of ovarian function. A woman who loses her ovaries at 30, has a similar degree of bone weakness when she turns 50, as a 70-year-old women who has gone through natural menopause.[14]

Also, the effectiveness of estrogen replacement therapy is directly related to how quickly it is begun after ovarian function declines. Lindsay and others have shown repeatedly, in long-term double-blind studies, that estrogen therapy begun immediately after ovarian loss, maintains bone at normal strength for decades. If estrogen therapy is begun years after ovarian loss, it maintains only the bone strength that still remains at that time.[15] The superiority of bone strength in women who begin estrogen replacement as soon as they lose ovarian function is shown in Figure 7 below.

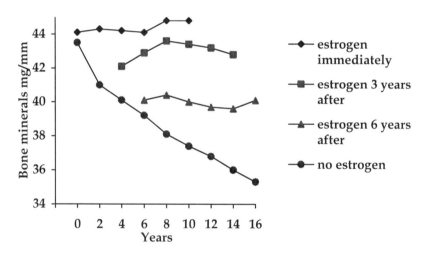

Figure 7. Long-term prevention of bone loss by estrogen. The earlier estrogen is begun after loss of ovarian function, the greater the bone mass retained. (Source: Lindsay et al, Reference 15.)

For women not butchered by surgery, it is vital to begin replacement therapy as soon as estrogen begins to decline. That is at perimenopause.[16] It's also vital to understand that once bone loss has occurred, estrogen alone will not rebuild it. Rebuilding lost bone requires estrogen, natural progesterone, and the nutrition and exercise program given above.

Don't leave anything to chance. Take this book and the medical references to your physician. Despite the whizbang surgery of hip replacement, which remains at best a hobble-de-hoy solution, most of your bones can't be replaced at all. It's the medicine man's job to protect them.

Estrogen Against Diabetes

While giving a paper on hormone replacement at the 1995 Convention of the American Academy of Anti-Aging Medicine, a sudden realization struck me dumb. Discussing the pathways by which insulin affects estrogen levels, I suddenly realized that they must be two-way paths. Estrogen levels must also affect insulin and glucose. Estrogen deficiency after menopause must raise insulin resistance and push women towards the diabetic end of the sugar control continuum. Loss of estrogen must increase the risk of adult-onset diabetes, and estrogen replacement should prevent it.

My mouth finished the lecture on automatic pilot, while my brain raced to get at the Internet medical libraries to look for evidence. I found only three studies, all very recent. In July 1990, in a study on heart disease, Dr. E. Barrett Conner at the University of California, San Diego compared the insulin levels of healthy postmenopausal women who were on estrogen or estrogen/progesterone, with postmenopausal women not taking these hormones. Those on hormone replacement showed much *lower* levels of insulin.[17] So far so good.

In September 1992, Dr. J. Manson and colleagues at Channing Laboratory in Boston, reported a huge 12-year study on the development of non-insulin dependent diabetes in 21,000 healthy women who went through either surgical or natural menopause. Those who used estrogen or estrogen/progesterone replacement, showed a much lower incidence of diabetes.[18] Better and better.

In October 1993 Dr. S Lindheim and colleagues at the University of Southern California, Los Angeles, tested the effects of estrogen on insulin metabolism in apparently healthy postmenopausal women. Three great findings. First, a whopping 44% of non-obese postmenopausal women showed the pre-diabetic syndrome of **insulin resistance**.

Second, moderate dose estrogen replacement (0.625mg/day Premarin) improved insulin sensitivity by 25% in only two months. As insulin becomes more sensitive, it takes less insulin in the blood to deal with blood sugar.

Third, high-dose estrogen (1.25mg/day Premarin) made insulin resistance *worse* by 25%. This evidence is the first demonstration that low-dose estrogen replacement may inhibit development of diabetes, and high-dose (excess) estrogen may accelerate diabetes. Keep in mind, its the *dose* that makes estrogen either a medicine or a poison.[19]

Estrogen Against Colon Cancer

It's common belief that breast and other reproductive system cancers of women are somehow matched by prostate and colo-rectal cancers of men. Our celestial maker, however, did not seem to have gender equality high on the list of design criteria. Women suffer many more reproductive system cancers than men, over 50,000 more cases in America every year.[20]

In addition, contrary to the notion that colon and rectal cancers are mainly male diseases, latest figures show that more women now develop colon cancer than men, and almost as many develop rectal cancer. With 74,000 new female cases out of 130,000 total new cases each year, an American woman's lifetime risk of colo-rectal cancer is a frightening 1 in 17.[20] Colo-rectal cancer has surged in incidence and severity to become America's second leading cause of cancer death.[21]

Estrogen therapy takes a big bite out of that risk. In a new study at the University of Wisconsin Medical School, researchers compared 694 postmenopausal women with colon or rectal cancer against 1600 healthy postmenopausal women. Use of estrogen replacement at any time in life, reduced the risk of colon cancer by 30%. Recent use of estrogen cut the risk almost in half.[22]

The largest ongoing study is the Cancer Prevention Study (CPSII), of 1,200,000 American men and women from all 50 states, begun by the American Cancer Society in 1982. Analysis of 422,000 postmenopausal women over the last 13 years, shows unequivocally that estrogen prevents many cases of colon cancer. In agreement with the Wisconsin study above, anytime use of estrogen replacement reduced the risk of fatal colon cancer by 30%. The longer the women used estrogen, the lower their risk became. Use for 11 years or more, halved the risk of fatal colon cancer.[23]

The reason estrogen inhibits colon cancer is likely the same reason it inhibits cardiovascular disease - reduction of cholesterol.[24] Cholesterol ends up as bile acids in the colon, an excess of which is linked to colon cancer.[25] Less cholesterol, less bile acids, less colon cancer, and probably less of a lot of other diseases, including gastrointestinal problems and gallstones.

These benefits alone make correct postmenopausal use of estrogen an enormous boon. And with a tip of my hat to comedians Fry and Laurie, we are always on the lookout for enormous boons.

Estrogen For Sex

Vaginal lubrication dries up with menopause. Even high sexual arousal cannot restore it. Intercourse often becomes an obstacle course of discomfort, pain, and frequent injury. Even if they stop sex altogether, many women still suffer vaginal burning, itching, irritation, and urinary dysfunction.[26]

Loss of vaginal structures supported by estrogen also raises the risk of uterine prolapse, as insufficient flesh and tone remains to support the uterus.[27] With uterine pressure, intercourse often becomes so uncomfortable it causes nausea, headache, and general loss of well-being for hours or even days afterwards.

In Sweden, research at the University Hospital in Linkoping by Dr. R. Lindgren and colleagues, found that one in every four postmenopausal women suffer such severe vaginal problems, they virtually terminate their sex life.[28] The worst of it is, sexual desire may continue. But, because of estrogen deficiency, fulfillment is denied.

Abstinence only compounds vaginal degeneration. Why? Dr. Wolf Utian, Professor of Reproductive Biology at Case Western Reserve University in Cleveland, recently stated the answer publicly to prudish America, which he rightly indicts as far behind Europe in recognizing women's problems. "Sexual intercourse itself helps maintain the machinery."[29]

Dr. Utian has been a world leader in menopause research for more than a quarter century. He started the International Menopause Society and its medical journal **Maturitas** in 1978. He knows what he's talking about. Use it or lose it.

Detrimental changes are not confined to the sex organs. Skin, breast and lip sensitivity frequently change so that once delightful kisses and caresses now produce only irritability.[30] One woman referred to the Colgan Institute describes it well, "I used to love my husband's hands on me. Now they feel like sandpaper. And his mustache used to give me goosebumps. Now - ugh!" With the right nutritional and multi-hormonal strategies, we returned the mustache to its former glory.

Dr. Lila Nachtigall of New York University Medical Center has followed women on estrogen and estrogen/ progesterone/testosterone therapy for many years. She reports that even women whose sex life is dormant, can be restored by replacement therapy. And even the worst cases of vaginal atrophy, often respond to topically applied estrogen creams.[16]

Other studies show that, many cases of vaginal atrophy can be reversed by estrogen pills,[31] with subsequent great sexual satisfaction. So for the sake of your health, your sex life, and even the feel of your skin, take these facts and the medical references to your physician.

A Woman's Eyes

Drying, thinning, and atrophy of the vagina and its support structures, are the best documented degenerative change in skin and mucous membranes that occur with menopause.[32] But many medicine men, who did their physiology training way back, seem to have forgotten that estrogen, progesterone, and testosterone support the skin and mucous membranes all over your body. These ubiquitous hormones maintain your mouth, gums, lips and eyes, and your entire suit of skin, plus the hair and nails that grow out of it.[5] When they decline at menopause, everything sags.

Wrinkles accelerate, hair thins, dries and coarsens, cheeks fall in, lips lessen, gums recede, nails talon, teeth yellow. Worst of all, eyes dry and fade, and sink into the sockets as they lose supporting tissue. Look around you.

Until now, hormone treatment to maintain beauty was thought trivial by medicine. Finally intelligence is prevailing. Physicians are coming to realize that good looks are linked inextricably to confidence, well-being, sexuality, and zest for life. Sophia Loren summed it up perfectly in a news interview for her role in the 1995 film *Grumpier Old Men*.

Looking elegant and beautiful in her 60s, she said, "It's a privilege to be seductive."

Estrogen Grows Collagen

With correct replacement therapy, most of the degenerative changes of menopause can be postponed for decades, some indefinitely. I have space to cite only a few recent studies. Let's look at **collagen**.

Collagen provides much of the supporting structure for your skin. Dry and thin postmenopausal skin and mucous membranes show massive collagen loss. New research shows that estrogen can prevent and even restore it.

In 1993, the Chelsea and Westminster Hospital in London, gave postmenopausal women estrogen implants to see if the therapy would reverse osteoporotic degeneration of their bones. To their delight, researchers found not only an increase in markers of bone strength, but also a rise in skin collagen throughout the body.[33]

A 1994 study provides further support. Postmenopausal women were treated for 12 months with estrogen at the St. Francis of Assisi Hospital in Quebec. Compared with a control group given placebo pills, skin thickness increased dramatically. With the blossom of new skin, the women also reported a new bloom in their quality of life.[34] By rejuvenating what these women saw in the mirror every day, estrogen also rejuvenated their whole mental outlook.

Estrogen Grows Elastin

New collagen restores structure, but what about skin elasticity, the spring-back quality of all young skin, largely conferred by the substance **elastin**. With menopause, skin elasticity vanishes faster than fairy dust.

In 1995, at the University of Liege in Belgium, menopausal women given estrogen, were compared with a control group of menopausal women, and with a group of perimenopausal women. Results showed a dramatic loss of skin elasticity during perimenopause and further losses with menopause. The women given estrogen, however, maintained the level of skin elasticity they had at the start of the treatment.[35] If you want to maintain skin tone and prevent your face and neck from sagging into age, the time to begin is at perimenopause.

Alas, despite all the face creams, you can't put collagen or elastin into your skin from the outside. They don't penetrate. Nor do they stay put, even if injected, as tens of thousands of women have sadly discovered. They have to grow from within. Getting the right hormones to the skin cells to stimulate new growth is the only way.

If women make sufficient noise, hormone creams which *do* penetrate skin will be quickly developed for general use. Local application of hormones will then replace the current witches brews of cosmetics. Estee Lauder and all the rest of the cosmetic houses will love the change, because they are the only folk who have the expertise and technical capacity to make the new creams. For the first time in cosmetic history they will have something that actually works.

From the latest research presented at the 1995 Conference of the Academy of Anti-Aging Medicine[36] and other 1995 scientific conferences on aging[37] I am confident that, once current research is incorporated into health-care, we will have women of 80 with the energy, physical capacity, and looks of 30. Best of all, this new evidence, which forms part of our **Hormonal Health Program,** will protect that wonderful luminous light that shines from a woman's eyes.

Estrogen Saves Jobs

The Mid-life Study at Yale University examines the effects of menopause on women's lives. The majority of menopausal women going through this research program without estrogen replacement therapy, show multiple menopausal symptoms that interfere with their careers and their ability to work.

In addition to hot flashes and other physical symptoms, most of these women suffer sleep disturbances, loss of memory, excessive worrying and anxiety, difficulty in concentrating, and loss of the ability to make decisions. One woman in every three suffers obsessive behavior, temper outbursts, and fear of leaving their home. All of these symptoms are promptly reduced or eliminated by estrogen therapy.

In taking the therapy, many of the women have saved their working careers. Researchers give examples of the banker whose hot flashes and palpitations prevented her carrying out business meetings, the opera singer whose anxiety attacks prevented her performing, and the teacher who could no longer bear her pupils to touch her. These women were restored to enjoying their careers by a simple increase in their estrogen levels provided by a little white pill.[38]

The number of otherwise healthy women forced to give up their work by menopause is unknown. But likely it's in the millions. To most folk work is vital, not only financially, but also as a source of satisfaction, confidence, and self-worth. In fact work is more than that. Numerous studies show that compared with homemakers, women with paid employment have higher self-esteem, less anxiety and depression, and better physical health.[39]

But those are only bland research findings of the value of work. More important are those essential effects of working that defy scientific measurement.   As a scientist I can approach them only through appeals to the spirit.

You Are What You Do

Labor is the thread
That weaves your hours into a symphony.
The melody created by your work
Defines life's purpose and directs life's course.

Therefore, love your labor, cherish it as a beloved.
Give to it from your heart and from your spirit.
Shape it in the likeness of your soul.
If you cannot, then 'tis better to be idle
Than weave your days into a misfortune and a dread.

As you fashion your labor, so it fashions you.
Strive for excellence in what you do,
And mastery will grow within your mind.
Strive for compassion every working day,
And love will blossom in your heart.
Strive for honor towards your fellow
And nobility will come to fill your soul.
Then the purpose of life is bound to your being
And its realization shines from your eyes.

Michael Colgan

From Colgan M, **Poems to Live By**, San Diego: CI Publications 1989.

Estrogen Extends Life

Studies of estrogen benefits in prevention of disease have hinted that women on estrogen replacement live longer. Cumulative analysis of all the major studies by Drs. Milton Weinstein and Anna Tosteson at Harvard University shows a strong trend towards extension of healthy life. The benefits to heart and bone of unopposed estrogen replacement for 5 years more than offsets any increased risk of cancer. Estrogen plus progestins gives even better life extension because it also eliminates most of the cancer risk. Estrogen plus progestins for 15 years extends life dramatically.[5]

Until now some scientists have questioned such meta-analyses as being a hodge-podge of too many disparate data. In 1996 everything changed. Dr. Bruce Ettinger provided direct evidence. Over many years he had been analyzing the medical histories of 454 women, born between 1900 and 1915, who were members of the Kaiser Permanente Medical Program. All were healthy in 1969. About half of them used estrogen replacement or had used it for at least one year. The death rate from all causes of the women who had not used estrogen was almost *double* that of the estrogen users.[41]

There is no longer any doubt that estrogen replacement, even in the crude form it is done today, can extend women's lives. When correct estrogen/progesterone/testosterone replacement is used as part of a full **Hormonal Health Program**, I predict the results will shatter current beliefs about the limits of human lifespan.

—— 14
Hormones Or Not

A common objection I get in lectures is: "I refuse to use hormones! They're unnatural, they're drugs. They can't be good for me."

That's about the same as refusing antibiotics for life-threatening infections, or refusing to get your children immunized against disease. It's a basic misunderstanding of our place in Nature and the crucial role of modern science in preventing illness.

We vainly think of ourselves as separate from the world, each somehow safe, untouched in our little skin bags. In truth we are just localized bits of the mass of liquids, solids and gases that whirls around us and through us every living day.

Our world, including us, is all one single system of chemistry. Science can track the course of these chemicals through the oceans, through the air, through the soil, through the plants and animals we eat, through our bodies, and back to the oceans again. To the extent that researchers discover how to adjust this flow of chemicals through our bodies, so as to retain the beneficial and discard the damaging, then we will live longer and healthier lives.

Because of recent discoveries about the loss of beneficial hormones with menopause, ten million American women are now retaining more estrogen, by putting supplements of the hormone into their bodies in the form of a pill.[1] The most common brand is **Premarin** which contains several forms of estrogen. Premarin is made from **PRE**gnant **MAR**e's ur**IN**e.[2] For women in my lectures who can't believe they have been swallowing horse pee, I crush a couple of Premarin pills and mix the powder in some warm water. The smell is unmistakable.

Those opposed to hormones or "unnatural" drugs may smile smugly as if I am supporting their viewpoint. On the contrary, I explain that the normal human diet contains many nutritious foods, that include all sorts of hormones. Such delicacies as Stilton cheese, lobster thermidor, crab bisque, oysters, deviled kidneys, and chicken a-la-king, all contain hormones and other drugs, built into them by Nature's design. Premarin is merely an extract from a natural, though not palatable, source.

Being vegetarian doesn't make any difference. Wheat contains opiate drugs.[3] Oatmeal contains a hormone that acts to release human luteinizing hormone.[4] "Good, wholesome" milk contains the hormones melatonin, and

growth-hormone-releasing-hormone.[5]   Active   hormones
enter your body in a whole host of foods.

Even the humble soybean contains **genistein** and other
estrogenic compounds.[6] One known effect of genistein is to
bind onto estrogen receptors, and thereby help control
estrogen.   The regular use of tofu, miso and other soy
products, is one reason why Asiatic women suffer fewer
menopausal problems than Western women, and have much
lower rates of breast and reproductive system cancers.[7,8]

You cannot avoid eating the multiple active drugs that are
part of the built-in design of your food. Once you realize
that hormones, drugs, nutrients, and foods are all parts of
the same single system of chemistry, then all the silly
arguments about "natural" versus "unnatural" evaporate for
the hot air they are.   The real question is: how much of
particular chemicals should I put into my body for hormonal
health?

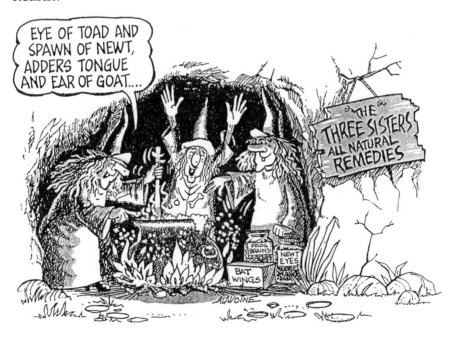

To simplify, I will divide this question into four parts:

1. What bodily hormones, and other chemicals can benefit human health when they are restored to youthful levels?

2. If the form of the chemical is a man-made derivative of a chemical that occurs in Nature, does it match the natural form sufficiently to be beneficial?

3. What are the beneficial dosages? Remember, it's the **dose** that makes a chemical either a benefit or a poison.

4. How can each appropriate chemical be delivered to sites of action in the body, in the right dose at the right time, so as not to disrupt the synchronized daily and monthly rhythms of thousands of other bodily chemicals?

The Hormonal Health Program

Numerous chapters in this book have shown you how the cascade of hormones from the pituitary gland in your brain, determines everything from your sexuality and emotions, your muscles and bones, to your intelligence and immunity. You have seen also how this cascade is orchestrated by the output of brain hormones and neurotransmitters in specific brain areas, primarily the striatal cortex and the hypothalamus. Researchers, including myself who are developing the **Hormonal Health Program**, realized over a decade ago, that in order to prevent degenerative changes in bodily hormones, we have to begin in the control center - the human brain.

Melatonin Supply

To follow the new therapy, you need to know about one other bit of your brain - **the pineal gland**. By its release of the hormone **melatonin**, this pea-sized master computer has now proved to be the controller of everything. Brilliant new research shows clearly, that if you want to compensate for the hormonal decline of usual aging, you better start with the pineal.[9]

Still referred to as the third eye, the pineal gland lies deep in your brain, as shown in Figure 8. It is turned on and off by the simplest and most ancient stimulus we know - light. Light entering your eyes, stimulates a bit of your hypothalamus called the **suprachiasmatic nucleus**. Lying just behind the eyes, this nucleus sends signals to the pineal gland. It also stimulates the preoptic nucleus of the

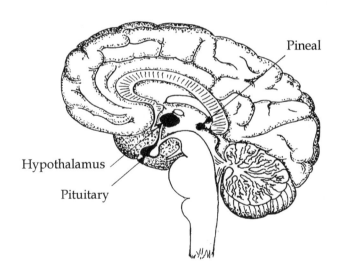

Figure 8. Midsection through brain showing pineal gland, hypothalamus, and pituitary.

hypothalamus, which I showed you in previous chapters, is the control center for human libido. Now you know why the sight of a good pair of buns can make your libido fire with enthusiasm.

The pineal gland, however, is concerned only with the *intensity* of light entering the eyes. During daylight, signals from the suprachiasmatic nucleus keep the pineal quiet. During the hours of darkness the pineal comes to life, releasing a big burst of melatonin, which synchronizes the circadian (24-hour) rhythm of your whole hormone cascade.[10]

Your melatonin supply declines rapidly with usual aging. As the primary controller, it is the first hormone that needs attention if you want to achieve hormonal health.

Dopamine And Acetylcholine

The initial trip down the hormone cascade from the pineal gland, lands you in the hypothalamus and striatal cortex. As we saw in earlier chapters, major controllers in these areas include the neurotransmitter systems for acetylcholine and dopamine. We saw also that these systems decline rapidly with usual aging.

Scientists have now isolated numerous chemicals that can inhibit these declines. One is the nutrient amino acid **acetyl-l-carnitine**, which we will see, can maintain acetylcholine function. Another is the chemical **selegiline**, which can maintain dopamine function. These chemicals are so important in maintaining your hormonal milieu against the ravages of aging, that I give each a separate chapter ahead.

Don't Mess With The Pituitary

Next port-of-call down the hormone cascade is your pituitary gland, which secretes a pile of intermediate hormones. Not a lot can yet be done to maintain pituitary function.

The most common pituitary problem is excess prolactin secretion, a potent disrupter of hormone balance. If you develop a *documented* case of excess prolactin, which is often caused by a slow-growing pituitary tumor, **bromocriptine** and other drugs can restore the balance. But don't let any anti-aging buffs, or their publications, talk you into bromocriptine as a general replacement therapy. It has numerous toxic and nasty side effects.[2]

In any case, the problem of increased prolactin secretion, and reduced output of other pituitary hormones, is often caused by reduced dopamine function back upstream at the striatal cortex. In the **Hormonal Health Program**, dopamine is the main focus of intervention to maintain the pituitary.

No Vasopressin

The pituitary hormone **vasopressin** deserves mention, because some previous popular books have recommended using an atomizer form (Diapid), to spray this hormone into your nose. The object is to stimulate brain function and sexuality, by absorption through the nasal epithelium (lining) straight into the hypothalamus.[11] Snorting cocaine works the same way.

Vasopressin, however, has multiple, complex effects at various points on the hormone cascade. No one has measured the long-term consequences of pumping it up your hooter whenever the fancy takes you. But, such a powerful hormone can change your body in all sorts of detrimental ways. Especially so, if it's out of synchrony with the levels or the rhythm of other hormones.[12] As a hands-on scientist, with no evidence of benefits to put my hands on, vasopressin is a definite no-no.

Growth Hormone: Rarely Useful

Lauded as the modern "Fountain of Youth", the pituitary hormone, **human growth hormone** has become a darling of the yuppie press. For many ailing aging, injections of growth hormone immediately fire up their lives. As we will see, however, this fire is soon extinguished. But ashes don't make good news copy, so the public continues to be misled.

With a new easy-to-use liquid form of growth hormone made by Genentech, and just approved by the FDA, this hormone is set to become a billion-dollar business in America by the year 2000. Despite its current FDA approval only to treat dwarfism, no regulation will be able to prevent the wealthy, aging mass of baby-boomers from getting their hands on it.

I would love to be able to tell you different, but all the growth hormone tales of anti-aging are just media flapdoodle. We include it as part of the **Hormonal Health Program** for two reasons. First, it has minor utility in some cases. Second, growth hormone is so falsely promoted and wildly abused in America today, that the scientific truth needs every public airing it can get. To prevent you or your physician being fooled, I give it a separate chapter ahead.

Dehydroepiandrosterone (DHEA):

The other downstream stop on the hormone cascade where replacement seems to make sense, concerns the pituitary hormone, **adrenocorticotrophic hormone (ACTH)**. ACTH travels from your pituitary to your adrenal glands, where it initiates the conversion of cholesterol into all your steroid hormones.[13] This conversion includes manufacture of a whole lot of intermediate hormones. One intermediate getting a lot of press is **dehydroepiandrosterone (DHEA)**.

DHEA is the most abundant steroid hormone in your body. Yet most of its precise functions remain unknown. Nevertheless, in long-term trials, DHEA has shown virtually zero toxicity. Studies report that it stimulates sexual function, improves well-being, lowers cholesterol, and boosts immunity.[14]

DHEA also declines reliably with usual aging in men, and abruptly in menopausal women.[14] Now it's being gobbled like candy as an anti-aging therapy. Not a good idea. I give DHEA a chapter ahead, which outlines a reasonable way to make use of it.

Testosterone: Sometimes

The testes are the end of the line in the male hormone cascade, at least it simplifies the chemistry to think of them that way. Testosterone is the usual end-organ hormone that physicians currently prescribe, all by itself, for aging men who show low testosterone levels, or complain of sexual problems or general debility. A very bad idea.

Much better is to give testosterone to menopausal women, to prevent the estrogen in female replacement therapy from running wild. But only the best physicians are yet aware of this benefit.

Willy-nilly use of testosterone by both men and women, has rocketed over the last five years, and will probably continue to rocket into the 21st century. Why? Because it has an immediate boosting effect on well-being and sexuality.

Alas, as you will see in the chapters ahead, the usual programs of testosterone replacement destroy all its benefits within a few months. Don't mess with testosterone until you know exactly what you are doing.

Estrogen and Progesterone: Yes

The other two end-organ hormones widely misused today are the various forms of estrogen, and progesterone (and its man-made mimics, progestins). As we will see in their chapters, the usual therapy is likely to cause more harm than good.

Don't fret, effective estrogen replacement therapy is just around the corner. Hopefully most physicians will soon come to know it. If you my readers disseminate the evidence in this book everywhere you go, it will cut years off this sorely needed medical transformation.

A Simple Strategy

The **Hormonal Health Program** may sound complex, but it's really simple. Your body ages from the brain down, from pineal control center down to end organs. To offset aging and degeneration of your hormonal system by replacement therapy, you therefore have to replace hormones from the brain down. Points of intervention and their hormones and other chemicals that we know most about are summarized in the table below.

The Hormonal Health Program Replacement Chemicals	
Point on Cascade	**Replacement Chemical**
Pineal gland	Melatonin
Hypothalamus	Selegiline
	Acetyl-l-carnitine
Pituitary	Growth hormone (GH)
Adrenals	Dehydroepiandrosterone (DHEA)
Testes	Testosterone
Ovaries	Estrogens
	Progesterone

Many other chemicals are used in anti-aging therapy. But, until you have a strategy that covers the above, plus a good nutrition and exercise program to support them, all others are secondary.

The basic principle of hormonal health is: **Never replace anything at any point on the hormone cascade, unless you ensure that controlling hormones and other chemicals further upstream have also been restored to youthful levels, so that they can work in synergy with the new downstream influx**.

Remember, the **Hormonal Health Program** is on the cutting edge of medical science. No extended human trials yet exist to prove its benefits. So before using any of these substances, take this book and the medical references to your physician. If he is unfamiliar with these developments, then find a physician who is.

The Colgan Institute does not administer hormone replacement programs. We are a research and consulting resource that provides the science to physicians and other health professionals. Your best bet for a knowledgeable physician is a member of the Academy of Anti-Aging Medicine. The phone number of their administration in Chicago is 312-248-8744.

15

Estrogen Therapy

The human body contains many kinds of estrogen. Those we know most about are **estradiol, estrone** and **estriol**. They form the estrogen component of the **Hormonal Health Program**.

In men, testosterone aromatizes (converts) to estrogens at various body sites, including the brain. In women the ovaries are the primary source. Because of ovarian decline, female estrogen levels begin to fall at perimenopause, usually between ages 40-45.[1]

Younger women who suffer hysterectomies, show an immediate estrogen decline whatever their age.[2] As you saw in the hysterectomy chapter, even women given the forms of surgery that conserve their ovaries, show detrimental changes in estrogen function.

In women, replacement therapy to maintain points on the hormone cascade upstream of the ovaries is insufficient. Intervention is still required at this end organ level, because of the primary ovarian decline that occurs both with natural menopause and with all forms of hysterectomy.

Estrogen Prescription: Rude and Crude

Current estrogen replacement therapy does not do the job. It uses primarily **conjugated equine estrogens** (**CEE**), with or without man-made progestins. Folk generally know CEE by the brand name, Premarin. Premarin contains estradiol, the strongest estrogen, plus estrone and estriol. These estrogens are pretty close to the human varieties, but *not* identical. Premarin also contains other horse estrogens, mainly **equilin** and **equilenin**, that don't occur in the human body.[3] No one knows what happens to them once they get inside you. But the biggest problem with CEE is not the hormone content, it's the way estrogen is prescribed.

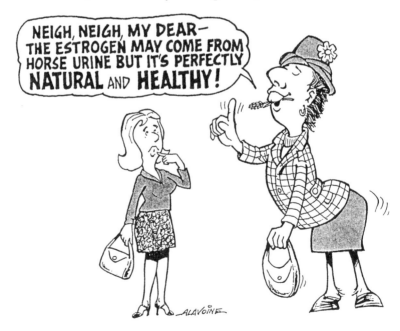

Remember, one principle of correct replacement therapy is to restore the hormone cascade to youthful levels. To do this optimally, you have to restore *each* person's *individual* youthful levels. The size and shape of your estrogen curve, is as individual to your body as the size and shape of your feet. I'm sure you know the painful results of shoes that don't fit. Current estrogen therapy is like forcing everyone to wear a size 9. The goal of the **Hormonal Health Program,** is to make your replacement therapy fit your body at least as well as your shoes fit your feet.

The normal range of individual differences in female estrogen levels is enormous. Some women are naturally low-estrogen, making only 50-200 micrograms of estrogen per day, depending on the phase of their menstrual cycle. To push them up near the top of the range with hormone replacement after menopause, is to court disaster and disease. Other women are naturally high-estrogen, making 100-700 micrograms of estrogen per day. To fail to get them back up to their natural level after menopause, allows menopausal decline to continue. Determining the correct dose is critical.

Most physicians, however, prescribe by seat-of-the-pants guesswork. They seem satisfied if the estrogen levels of their patients rise quickly to anywhere in the normal range, and their menopausal symptoms abate. This usually means a daily estrogen pill of 0.625mg, 1.25mg, or more.

For the majority of women, these doses of estrogen are way too high. Breast cancer specialist Dr. Susan Love was not exaggerating when she said: "Many gynecologists are handing out these hormones like M&Ms."[4] The excess estrogen works mischief throughout your body. The mischief is made all the worse by the failure of physicians to restore other points on the hormone cascade.

No wonder we see reports that women are sick all the time they are on estrogen.[5] No wonder that numerous women's groups reject hormone replacement altogether.[2] No wonder that doctors who have to treat estrogen-caused diseases are against it. Acquainting your physician with the medical studies reviewed in this book, could save you becoming one of the victims.

Measuring Your Estrogen Need

As more and more medicine men become aware of the new science, prescribed estrogen doses are falling in America.[2] That's a blessing. But the methods of calculating a woman's estrogen needs, are still not based on her youthful estrogen levels. If you have the medical records of your estrogen levels at age 20 - 25, take them to your physician as a basis for planning replacement. If you don't have the records, then get them by hook or by crook. They are the only accurate basis for planning replacement therapy.

If you simply can't get the records, then ensure that your physician uses at least the following criteria:

1. **Heart Protection**. The minimum estrogen dose
    that raises protective HDL cholesterol and
    lowers damaging LDL cholesterol, and thereby
    reduces the risk of cardiovascular disease.

2. **Breast Protection**. The estrogen dose that is unlikely to cause breast or reproductive system cancers.

3. **Bone Protection**. The minimum estrogen dose that prevents bone loss.

Combined, these three criteria to protect your heart, breasts, and bones, yield reasonable doses for two-thirds of menopausal women. Prior to menopause, their estrogen levels would have been in the middle of the youthful range.

For the scientists among you, these combined criteria yield a reasonable estrogen dose for about 68% of women (one standard deviation either side of the mean). But they are unlikely to meet the needs of the other 32%, who were naturally either low-estrogen or high-estrogen. In the absence of records of a women's youthful estrogen levels, they are the best science can do.

Many physicians do not have even these guides, or use only one of them, often based on only one or two studies. In designing the **Hormonal Health Program**, I and my colleagues have analyzed all studies to date to provide you with more accurate information.

Estrogen Dose For Heart Health

To estimate the estrogen dose required to give you cardiovascular protection, first we reviewed all major studies of oral CEE where dosage was known.[6-13] We had to use the CEE data, because most studies to date are of women on this form of replacement. We sought to determine the minimum dose of CEE that afforded the greatest rise in protective HDL cholesterol, and the greatest fall in detrimental LDL cholesterol.

One fly in the ointment is **triglycerides**, blood fats. In excess, triglycerides are a proven cardiovascular risk. High doses of estrogen replacement that often raise HDL cholesterol the most, also raise triglycerides the most. So we took the change in triglyceride levels into account, and devised a computer model to assess the dosage yielding greatest overall cardiovascular protection.

Surprise, surprise. CEE doses of only 0.33mg per day raised HDL cholesterol as much or more than doses of 1.25mg. They also lowered LDL cholesterol by similar amounts. But the low doses raised damaging triglycerides by only 1.5%, compared with 33% for the 1.25mg dose.

These data suggest that a CEE dose of only 0.33mg per day, affords *better* cardiovascular protection for postmenopausal women than any higher dose. You don't need much estrogen for your heart's sake, less than half the amount now prescribed to most women on hormone replacement. That's great news, because to continue to protect your body from menopausal decline, you need to take estrogen from perimenopause on.

Estrogen Dose To Avoid Breast Cancer

To estimate the best dose of estrogen to avoid breast cancer, we used the work of Dr. Louise Brinton at the U.S. National Cancer Institute, plus the research of Dr. Anne Paganini-Hill and others.[14-17] Breast cancer is a lifetime risk, so we had to assess both dosage and the change in risk with duration of estrogen use.

Results showed that a daily dose of 0.3mg of CEE, taken for 12.5 years by menopausal women who have avoided hysterectomies, does *not* increase the risk of breast cancer. In contrast, a daily dose of 1.25mg of CEE, increases breast cancer risk immediately by about 20%, and, after 10 years use, by about 75%. **Current research figures on estrogen and breast cancer, support a low estrogen dose (0.3mg/day) for long-term hormone replacement.**

Estrogen Dose To Save Your Bones

Assessing the dose of estrogen sufficient to prevent bone loss is difficult, because estrogen alone will not do it. Prevention of osteoporosis requires progesterone, the correct diet, and exercise as well. Also, most people with bone loss, do not go to their physician until the disease is far enough advanced to produce symptoms. So intervention is usually begun much too late to restore normal bone strength.

Certain characteristics of women also greatly affect risk of bone loss. As I show in my book, **The New Nutrition**, those who are naturally thin and small-breasted, or are smokers, or regular users of antacids, or have low levels of estrogen to begin with, or take a lot of caffeine, in coffee, tea, cola, etc., or are sedentary, all require strong intervention to save their bones.[18]

Nevertheless, our analysis of hundreds of case studies over the past decade, plus all major controlled studies, suggests that, **CEE doses of 0.2-0.6mg per day, combined with**

progesterone and the nutrition and exercise program given in Chapters 24 and 25, can stop further loss of bone and can increase bone strength. To be optimally effective, you need to start the whole program at perimenopause.

Too Much Estrogen

Calculating estrogen need by the three criteria, cardiovascular health, breast cancer prevention, and maintenance of bone, yields on average CEE dose of only 0.35mg per day. Most women now on estrogen replacement are given double or quadruple that amount. Our analysis of all major studies, suggests that disease and disorder resulting from CEE therapy, is not caused by estrogen replacement per se, nor by the form of estrogen, but by the excess doses of estrogen employed.

You can monitor whether or not you are getting too much estrogen by watching for some simple signs. The obvious one is growth of breast tissue, which causes breast tenderness and visible enlargement. Loss of frontal and crown head hair, intolerance of contact lenses, grey-brown blotches on facial skin, headache, dizziness and confusion are other good signs. If you get them, consult your physician to reduce your estrogen dose, or switch you to a form of estrogen from a different source.

The main types of estrogen used in America are listed in table below. Some popular articles mistakenly call some brands incomplete because they don't contain all three major estrogens, estradiol, estrone and estriol. Not so. In the human body, estradiol and estrone are constantly interconverted to maintain an equilibrium of circulating estrogens. Conversion of either to estriol also occurs freely and is final. That is, estriol cannot be converted back to other estrogens. So any brand that contains estradiol *or* estrone, provides the base for all three major forms of estrogen.

Forms of Estrogen Used For Hormone Replacement		
Brand Name	**Estrogens**	**Source**
Premarin (Wyeth-Ayerst)	Estradiol Estrone Estriol Equilin* Equilenin*	Pregnant mare's urine
Menest (SmithKline Beecham)	Estrone 75-85% Equilin* up to 15%	Pregnant mare's urine
Estratab (Solvay)	Estrone 75-85% Equilin* up to 15%	Pregnant mare's urine
Ogen (Upjohn)	Estrone	natural source
Orthoest (Ortho)	Estrone	natural source
Estrace (Bristol-Myers)	Estradiol	---
* Horse estrogens		

Source: Physician's Desk Reference, Reference # 3

If 0.35mg represents the average daily dose of estrogen required for long-term use, then the dosage range that would include most women is 0.10 - 0.60mg. When programs like the **Hormonal Health Program** come into general use, I predict that even these doses will prove too high, because correcting other points on the hormone cascade upstream of the ovaries, itself increases natural estrogen levels.

Estrogens that better match a woman's natural supply will further increase the benefits of replacement. Read on to discover the forms and combinations of estrogen that many women are calling "a rejuvenation miracle."

"Natural" Estradiol

Media reports lately have panned the horse estradiol in CEE in favor of estradiol from wild yams, especially *Diascorea composita*. Because of its vegetable origin, yam estradiol is often described as "natural and safe." In truth, it's a lot less natural than CEE. Yam estradiol is purely a man-made synthetic drug.

Wild yams contain negligible amounts of estrogen. But they are loaded with hormone precursors. By complex chemical wizardry, these precursors are transformed into synthetic estradiol, synthetic estrone, synthetic estriol, synthetic progesterone, synthetic testosterone and numerous other hormones.[19] They are about as natural as a polystyrene cup.

It's that silly natural versus unnatural argument again. The public have been so misled to believe yam estrogens are natural, that snake-oil merchants of the medical fringe have flooded the market with useless yam pills, yam potions, and yam creams, all touted to provide hormone replacement. Don't be fooled. The human body doesn't contain the necessary chemicals to effect the transformation of yam material into estrogens. And nothing known to science can do the job either, when added to any yam concoction that goes in or on your body.

The synthetic man-made estrogens from yams, however, sport a chemical difference from horse estrogens that makes them better and safer. They have been made by chemistry to be molecularly identical to human estrogens. Their chemical keys are an exact fit to the locks of your estrogen receptors.

Because of this smooth fit, yam-derived synthetic estrogens are likely to be more effective than equine estrogens. The difference is difficult to estimate because human data are lacking. From the limited evidence we have been able to gather at the Colgan Institute, the required daily dose of yam-derived estradiol or estrone is likely only 0.1-0.5 milligrams. That's 100-500 micrograms, less than half the usual dose of equine estrogens.

The Estriol Enigma

Estriol is the weakest of the three common forms of estrogen. It is formed in the body as an end metabolite of estradiol. Discovered way back in 1930, it's an age-old treatment for menopausal symptoms. The big advantage of estriol is, it does **not** cause wild cell growth in the female reproductive system, so does not raise the risk of cancer.[20,21] Better, estriol even appears to protect the body against cancerous changes in the breast and reproductive system caused by estradiol. Estriol reduces the binding of estradiol to cells where it can cause wild growth.[20]

Why estriol fell out of favor when more potent forms of estrogen were pushed into the marketplace, remains a mystery. I suspect profits and politics, but cannot find any evidence. One possibility is that physicians may have found estriol ineffective in America because of our high fat diet. High fat foods can inactivate oral estriol.[22] With the new American consciousness for lower fat diets, estriol should rise again to prominence.

There's no doubt estriol is effective. A recent five-year multi-center trial in Germany, showed that oral estriol succinate at 2.0-8.0mg per day, eliminated menopausal complaints and prevented vaginal atrophy. Side-effects were negligible.[21]

A new double-blind study at the Great Wall Hospital in Beijing, China, reports that a dose of only 2.0mg of estriol, given once every two weeks for a year, prevented bone loss. This very low dose also increased HDL cholesterol after six months treatment, thereby yielding cardiovascular protection too.[23]

Estriol sounds like the ideal estrogen: no cancer risk, elimination of menopausal complaints, protection of breasts, bones, and heart. Nevertheless I don't recommend estriol by itself as estrogen replacement. It is not convertible back to estradiol and estrone in the human body. So estriol alone cannot replace youthful estrogen levels, which consist primarily of estrone sulfate circulating in the bloodstream as a reserve pool, balanced roughly 50:50 with circulating estradiol. To replace estrogen properly you have to include some estradiol, and ideally, some estrone too.

The Tri-Est Formula

Brilliant physician Dr. Jonathan Wright of Kent, Washington, has popularized a combination of the three estrogens called Tri-Est, that fits the bill nicely. A typical Tri-Est pill is 2.0mg estriol, 250 micrograms estradiol, and 250 micrograms estrone.

Though not an approved combination yet in America, Tri-Est is readily available from Europe and by prescription from compounding pharmacies, such as The Women's International Pharmacy in Madison, Wisconsin, 1-800-279-5708. Your medical insurance should cover it.

You may need a higher dose of Tri-Est for acute menopausal complaints. But for long-term use, especially in combination with other parts of the **Hormonal Health Program**, as little as half the above dose may be ample.

Numerous women who have consulted the Colgan Institute to provide their physicians with this information, have adopted Tri-Est, in conjunction with a good nutrition regimen and other parts of the **Hormonal Health Program**. These are simple strategies. It doesn't take a rocket scientist to understand why they work. Nevertheless, against the present morass of health-care failure in America, we get to hear the word "miracle" fairly often nowadays.

16

Progesterone Wins

Estrogen is the dominant female hormone during the first half of a woman's menstrual cycle. **Progesterone** becomes dominant during the second half of the cycle. In mid-cycle, when the egg is released from the ovary, the corpus luteum (yellow body) forms and releases progesterone. Progesterone then triggers changes in the lining of the womb to prepare it for pregnancy. Progesterone also inhibits the action of estrogen, which otherwise would stimulate the immune system to destroy a fertilized egg as a foreign body. This progesterone miracle of protection, without which we would not exist, goes on every month of a fertile woman's life. Progesterone is the primary control agent that keeps estrogen in line.

At perimenopause everything changes. As estrogen levels begin to fluctuate and lose synchronicity, so do progesterone levels. Research in New Zealand shows that the number of ovulatory cycles declines by 40% during perimemopause.[1]

The progesterone phase of the menstrual cycle also becomes shorter.[2]   Together, these phenomena reduce female progesterone levels dramatically.

After menopause it gets worse. The research of Dr. Christopher Longcope at the University of Massachusetts shows that, on cessation of menstrual cycles, a woman loses two-thirds of her remaining progesterone. Within six months blood levels decline from a viable 1.60 ng/ml to a barely functional 0.5 ng/ml.[3]

Despite these clear findings, current health authorities have no policy to restore progesterone. It beats me that they are then surprised when estrogen replacement runs wild. Obscure rationalizations flow back and forth across the medical journals that remind me of talks between Eeyore and Piglet.   No one is listening and no one is home. Meanwhile, millions of women suffer.

The Progestin Deception

It's a medical disgrace that the 1996 **Physicians Desk Reference** contains no progesterone for hormone replacement. Pharmaceutical companies refuse to sell it because, as a naturally occurring chemical, they can't patent it. Instead they have invented profitably patentable **progestins**, also called **progestogens**, man-made mimics of progesterone that never existed in Nature, and have no natural place in a woman's body.[4]

Some physicians make no distinction between progesterone and progestins. They even seem to think that progestins are an "improvement" on progesterone. Such arrogance! If you are concerned to achieve hormonal health, always, always realize the clear distinction between molecules that form part of Nature's magnificent design, and molecules made by the puny hand of man.

Progestins do perform some of the functions of progesterone. They prevent overgrowth of the endometrium, for example, by causing the wild cells to shed. That's why they are added to estrogen replacement therapy, to prevent endometriosis and subsequent endometrial cancer. All well and good, but the chemical keys of man-made progestins don't fit the locks of Nature, so they cause all sorts of trouble elsewhere.

As part of this trouble the **Physicians Desk Reference** cites breast cancer, birth defects, strokes, and a variety of lesser ills.[4] Despite these detrimental effects, progestins have received little research attention or public scrutiny. They are prescribed freely, yet another example of the hormonal mistreatment of women. The evidence that we do have on progestins does not recommend them at all. Let's look at a couple of pertinent examples.

Progestins Increase Heart Risk

Synthetic progestins come in two main forms, 19-nortestosterones and 17-hydroxyprogesterones. The most common 19-nortestosterone products are **norethindrone** and **levonorgestrel**. They come under multiple brand names. As their testosterone source implies, both have strong androgenic (masculinizing) side-effects. And any hormone that makes the female system more male, likely increases the risk of heart disease.

We saw in earlier chapters how estrogen replacement reduces a woman's risk of heart disease by increasing her protective HDL cholesterol. But if you add either of the above progestins, in doses sufficient to prevent the endometriosis induced by estrogen replacement, this heart protection is eliminated. Whether given alone or in conjunction with estrogen, both norethindrone and levonorgestrel reduce HDL by 20 - 30%. Such a reduction puts your whole cardiovascular system in jeopardy.[5-7]

The most common of the second type of progestins, and the most frequently prescribed of all, is **medroxyprogesterone**. It comes in multiple brands too. As its progesterone source implies, medroxyprogesterone is only mildly androgenic. Nevertheless, in doses sufficient to prevent estrogen-induced endometriosis, it reduces HDL by about 16% when used alone, and by 8% when used with estrogen.[5-7] These changes may seem small, but HDL is only one measurement of increased cardiovascular risk. **The Physicians Desk Reference** issues strident warnings about blood clots, cerebral thrombosis, and pulmonary embolism under every listing for medroxyprogesterone.[4]

Natural progesterone causes no such cardiovascular problems. Doses sufficient to control the endometrial damage caused by estrogen replacement (200 mg/day), have no detrimental effects on HDL.[7] Dr. Joel Hargrove, Director of the PMS and Menopause Clinic at Vanderbilt University in Nashville, Tennessee, has been prescribing large doses of oral progesterone (300 - 500 mg per day) for the past 13 years. He has found no bad effects on the heart, the arteries, or any other part of the body.[8]

Why is progesterone so benign? Because its chemistry fits your chemistry. To quote Hargrove: "It doesn't fight with Mother Nature." For your heart's sake, natural progesterone is a clear winner over synthetic progestins.

Progestins Whack Emotions

Medical scientists have known about the emotional horrors of progestins since the mid '60s, when they were first added to estrogen to prevent endometrial cancers caused by the early contraceptives. But it was difficult to get funding for research likely to damn progestins, because they profitably prevented cancer, and without them the contraceptive industry was doomed.

Drug industry watchdogs, however, were not quite as vigilant as those of the tobacco industry, and some research slipped through into the medical literature. It showed clearly that progestins, especially the 19-nortestosterones, disrupt hormonal and emotional equilibrium to cause a sort of roller-coaster of alternating anxiety and depression.[9,10]

Progestins, especially medroxyprogesterone, are also notorious for causing irregular menstrual bleeding, bloating, and breast tenderness. Not the sort of effects that put anyone in a good mood.[11]

In contrast, natural progesterone has calming, even sedative effects on brain function.[12] Veterinarians often use progesterone implants on mares in hunting, show-jumping, and cross-country riding, because it keeps them calm, reduces the tendency to shy, and reduces horse premenstrual syndrome.

In women progesterone has been used successfully to treat premenstrual syndrome since the 1950s, when British physician Dr. Katherina Dalton first showed that PMS is a hormonal disorder.[13] Correctly given, progesterone eliminates the anxiety, irritability and depression common to premenstrual syndrome.[14] The only side-effects are beneficial - increased libido and euphoria.

Multiple Benefits of Progesterone

I could fill this book with the documented benefits of natural progesterone and the documented dangers of man-made progestins. But a few more examples will have to suffice. Dr. John Lee in California has shown repeatedly how the body can convert progesterone to numerous other hormones and biochemicals as needed, including testosterone. The natural hormone has all the chemical keys to fit exactly into the sequence of the hormone cascade. Because they lack many of these keys, your body cannot convert progestins into anything useful.[15]

One clear example of progesterone's wide-ranging functions is the reproductive cycle. During pregnancy, the placenta manufactures 20 times or more the normal level of progesterone in a woman's body. One major reason it does so, is to damp down estrogen's potentiation of her immune system. Otherwise estrogen dominance would cause the fetus to be rejected as a foreign body. Now you know why progesterone injections are often used to prevent miscarriages.

It's old medicine. I'm indebted to my friend, renowned British writer Leslie Kenton, for introducing me to the fascinating history of progesterone.[16] Medieval midwives used to use mistletoe berries to prevent miscarriage, because mistletoe, properly grown and gathered, contains effective levels of natural progesterone. Kissing under the mistletoe at Christmas derives from an ancient Druidic fertility festival, in which both men and women danced under the mistletoe, and drank honey mead laced with crushed mistletoe berries, -- and begat many children.

I wouldn't advise it though. Mistletoe also contains digitalis and other acutely toxic drugs. The old witches knew how to prepare it safely. We don't.

The extremely high levels of progesterone produced naturally during pregnancy have no toxicity at all. On the contrary, they benefit the woman in multiple ways. The fresh bloom of pregnancy that makes her look so good, for example, is a rejuvenative effect of progesterone on the skin.

In contrast to progesterone's complex chemistry which protect the mother and the growing fetus, man-made progestins are likely to damage both. Progestins carry warnings that their use during pregnancy is contraindicated for a variety of reasons, one of which is *double* the risk of certain birth defects.[4]

Progesterone For Bones

A final example of progesterone's benefits is bone. We have seen in earlier chapters how estrogen prevents bone loss. But, by itself estrogen *never* causes bone regrowth. As I explained, to get bone regrowth you have to add correct nutrition and weight-bearing exercise. Another little secret of the **Hormonal Health Program** is to add a little natural progesterone.

Your physician may not know this because it is not yet an approved therapy, but progesterone potentiates bone growth.[17,18] Man-made progestins do not. I will not burden you with the complex chemistry. Simply take the medical references to your physician. For your skeleton's sake, I hope they open his eyes.

Ditch Progestins

After analyzing all the available research, I have to conclude that there is no scientific reason to use man-made progestins in place of the natural progesterone molecule. But progestins are so obscenely profitable, that pharmaceutical companies can afford to employ armies of tame scientists to write reams of bogus justifications, defending them against any criticism. Pre-publication pieces from this book have already been criticized by physicians with high-sounding titles from apparently respectable universities. Uninformed media reporters naively accept such credentials as proof of wisdom. And the public continues to be misled.

Don't make the same mistake. Science is a system of evidence that owes no allegiance to title or position. If you doubt my conclusions, I ask only that you read the scientific references given, before you decide who is right.

Dosage and Timing

Progesterone is difficult to dissolve, so absorption via the oral route is very unreliable. In an attempt to overcome this problem, the hormone is pulverized into the finest of powders, called **micronized progesterone.** But most of it is still destroyed or excreted, either directly or in its first pass through the liver. Sublingual progesterone pellets or oils overcome this problem, but are not yet available to most folk. There is a much better way.

Progesterone in a moisturizing cream base is easily absorbed through the skin. No commercial products are available yet, but compounding pharmacies can make the cream on prescription from your physician. It works a treat.

Sensing the growing demand, numerous companies in the nutrient supplement and cosmetics industries, have flooded the market with creams containing **diosgenin** from the wild yam species *Diascorea*, and extracts of black cohosh, fenugreek, and other herbs that contain steroid precursors of progesterone. They are all bogus. The human body does not have the enzymes necessary to convert vegetable steroids into progesterone, and the amount of actual progesterone in these plants is negligible.[19]

It's true that progesterone is made commercially from the diosgenin of wild yams, but your body can't perform that chemistry. A good job too, otherwise your hormone balance would be at the mercy of the hundreds of plant steroids in our normal daily food.

Because the progesterone in prescription creams enters your bloodstream directly, and dodges the first pass through your liver, you need much less of the hormone via the skin route. The minimum effective dose of oral micronized progesterone is 200 mg per day. In a cream you need only 25 mg per day. The low dose is the way to go.

Progesterone is best absorbed through the thin skin areas of your body, those without much underlying fat. The face is ideal, followed by the upper back and chest (not the breasts), then arms and legs. Last preference is belly and hips.

Some physicians advise postmenopausal women to cycle the progesterone, two weeks on, two weeks off, to mimic the rhythm of their former menstrual cycle. This is a sensible strategy only if you are also cycling estrogen. It makes no sense to cycle progesterone, if you are using estrogen every day and no longer have a menstrual cycle.

No studies yet exist on cycled estrogen/progesterone therapy. But cycled estrogen/progestin therapy causes multiple side-effects in menopausal women. In contrast, continuous estrogen/progestin therapy shows few side-effects and good compliance.[20] Using progesterone instead of progestins should show even better results. Especially so if you use the **Hormonal Health Program** to maintain the rest of your hormone cascade.

Vary the site of progesterone application, because the skin and underlying dermis become saturated within a few days. You should welcome this progesterone saturation, long a beauty secret of cosmeticians to the stars. It stimulates skin collagen growth and growth of new blood vessels. When your friends remark how radiant you look, you are doing it right.

The benefit to skin, your largest organ, reflects similar benefits to every organ inside you. They continue as long as you continue to use progesterone. Numerous women on nutrition programs from the Colgan Institute have adopted progesterone cream as their lifelong moisturizer. It's as easy and harmless to use as your toothpaste, and does a great deal more for your health than polishing the pearly whites.

——17

Melatonin: Top Dog

Recent media reports applaud **melatonin** as a natural sleeping pill, and a way to beat jet lag. True enough, but these are only minor reflections of its functions. We know now that deficiency of pineal melatonin disrupts your hormones, your cognition, your immune system and your emotions. Melatonin deficit also increases your risks of cancer, cardiovascular disease, senility and a host of other disorders. When your melatonin runs down, everything goes.

I can't cover the mass of new studies here, but if you doubt me, Dr. Russell Reiter, Professor of Neuroendocrinology at The University of Texas, San Antonio, has just published an easy-reading, 250-page summary of the evidence.[1] That should be enough to convince you.

The Aging Clock

What you need to know here, is that pineal output of melatonin declines rapidly with usual aging. This decline is so reliable that numerous researchers now refer to the pineal gland as "The Aging Clock."[2]

I constructed the figure below from an average of all the major studies. In your mid-twenties peak nighttime melatonin output is about 50pg/ml. By age 30 it declines to 40pg/ml. By age 50 it drops to less than half the youthful level. By age 70, it's down to 10pg/ml, only 20% of the melatonin you have in your twenties. That's why a lot of old folk don't sleep well: they have insufficient melatonin.[2]

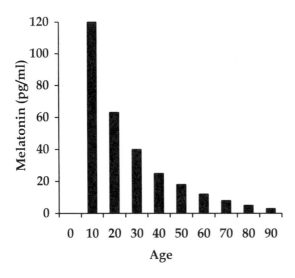

Figure 9. Nocturnal melatonin levels decline with usual aging.
Source: Colgan Institute, San Diego, CA

The first thing to do to inhibit aging of your whole hormonal system, is to restore the melatonin output of the master controller - the pineal gland. Without sufficient melatonin to direct the synchrony of your other hormones, you have little chance of getting them back into balance.

Most dangerous are the end-organ hormones at the bottom of the cascade, androgens and estrogens. They act directly on tissue to cause growth, therefore require the greatest control. With current hormone replacement, that vital control is non-existent. Many physicians, for example, restore female estrogen to youthful levels, without restoring melatonin or any of the other controllers further upstream. By doing so, they are putting in a powerful growth chemical with freedom to run wild. No surprise that it eventually causes enough wild growth to turn to cancer in the breasts and reproductive organs.

Benefits of Melatonin Replacement

Besides restoring the circadian synchrony of your hormones, many new studies show further benefits of melatonin. First, it is a powerful brain antioxidant that inhibits brain aging by destroying free radicals. These are damaging oxidation chemicals that are produced by toxins such as alcohol, and by normal brain metabolism of oxygen.[3]

Like James Bond in *Never Say Never*, you may refuse to give up your daily martini to avoid the free radicals from the liquor. By destroying them, melatonin could save your mind.

Melatonin may also act as a bodily antioxidant to prevent cancer.[4] It also boosts immunity against numerous other diseases, including AIDS.[2] It also helps to lower cholesterol and protect your heart.[2] It gives you better sleep and rest,[5] and it slows the decline in growth hormone that occurs with usual aging.[6]

Nutritional Melatonin

If you can't abide the thought of taking nightly pills, then go for night-time snacks of foods high in melatonin. Best sources are slow-cooking rolled oats, whole brown rice, and sweet corn, which contain 20-50mcg of melatonin per ounce. Bananas and tomatoes contain about half as much. New studies report that feeding animals such high melatonin foods increases their melatonin levels.[2]

Supplementing your diet with 500-1000mg of calcium also increases melatonin levels.[2] You should have at least this amount in your daily multi-vitamin/mineral. It has a larger effect on melatonin production when taken at night.

Vitamins B$_3$ (niacin) and B$_6$ (pyridoxine) affect melatonin too.[7] Other B vitamins and other essential nutrients are also likely to have a hand in the process, because all vitamins and minerals work in synergy with each other.[8] But the studies have not yet been done. Until scientists have had time to document the precise interactions, a **complete** multi-vitamin/mineral supplement provide sensible nutrition insurance for melatonin maintenance.

You can't do it with food alone. My book **The New Nutrition,** reviews the evidence that you cannot get sufficient vitamins and minerals from even a carefully chosen diet today. It discusses your needs for these nutrients in detail.[9] The best I can do in the space available here, is give you a formula in the Nutrition chapter which covers the needs of most folk.

Dose and Timing

Taking melatonin in a sublingual pill is the best way. It's not expensive - yet. Nor do you need much. No one knows the ideal dose, but 1.0 - 12.0 mg per night covers most people. I take 3 mg which seems sufficient to peak my nighttime melatonin levels near those of an average 25-year-old. My colleagues and clients take anywhere from 0.5 mg to 15.0 mg. In eight years of using melatonin in these doses, we have no reports of side-effects.

By usual toxicological tests, toxicity of melatonin is extremely low. Even doses of several hundred milligrams produce nothing more than sleepiness.[2] But no one knows the invisible long-term effects of large doses, subtle effects that must interfere with bodily processes. We know that excess melatonin can disrupt the hormone cascade, because high doses make a reliable contraceptive.[2] For replacement purposes, a few milligrams per night is plenty.

Timing is essential to avoid disrupting the synchrony of the hormone cascade. We take melatonin so that its presence in the bloodstream will coincide as far as possible with the natural nocturnal burst of the hormone. This burst occurs from about 1 am to 4 am in folk who keep usual sleep hours.[2] Western Society generally goes to bed around 10:30 pm or 11:30 pm, depending on which TV news offends least.

To allow for digestion and entry into the brain, we take melatonin one hour before accustomed bedtime.

Before you consider taking melatonin, take this book and the medical references to your physician. If he seems skeptical of melatonin's control over your hormone cascade, or says that melatonin supplements are unnecessary for hormone replacement, suspect a closed mind. You may want to find someone else to care for your health, who is better versed in recent medical science.

18

Selegiline For Life

Over the last decade, **selegiline hydrochloride** has become the dominant cognition-enhancing, hormone-potentiating, anti-aging compound in Europe.[1] There it is freely available under the brand names Deprenyl or Jumex.

Selegiline is fast gaining similar status in America, though it wasn't approved by the FDA until June 1989. Even then, approval under the name deprenyl (Eldepryl), was restricted to a minor adjunctive treatment to L-dopa therapy for Parkinson's disease.[2]

Thereby hangs a tale health authorities don't want you to know about. Despite restrictive approval, your physician can prescribe selegiline for hormone replacement, or for any other condition he deems fit. Health authorities control drug approvals. But once drugs are in the **Physicians Desk Reference**, physicians control prescription.

Pharmaceutical companies are a lot smarter than the regulators. They know that even the tiniest, most innocuous approval opens the prescription flood gates. The American Medical Association reports that up to half of all prescriptions are for non-approved uses.[3] Drug manufacturers aim their applications to the FDA accordingly. For a drug like selegiline, with multiple uses, and billion-dollar potential, they would have accepted an approval to treat warts.

In Britain, for example, selegiline was approved in October 1982.[1] Within five years it became the largest-selling product of Forum Holdings, the British license holder.

Remember most use of selegiline is happening against the stated policy of health authorities. The official position is that any compound that can improve brain function and emotions in folk with no medical condition, should be tightly controlled as a potential drug of abuse. As we will see, it is the health policy that abuses public well being rather than selegiline.

How Does It Work?

Selegiline is yet another derivative of **phenethylamine**, the base structure of many man-made stimulants and anti-depressants. Phenethylamine is a natural chemical widely distributed in humans, animals, and plants. It has multiple, strong effects on your body and brain. Phenethylamine is the chemical in chocolate that makes it such an addictive substitute for sex and affection.

Your body makes many essential biochemicals out of phenethylamine every day. Millions of derivatives are possible, each with unique biochemical activity. Selegiline may well be one of them that your body makes less and less efficiently with usual aging.

By this point in the book, you know that the decline of the neurotransmitter dopamine with usual aging, causes a downstream decline in the whole hormone cascade. Selegiline works by increasing active dopamine levels.

Selegiline also increases activity of the neurotransmitter norepinephrine.[4] Dopamine stimulates sexual desire, but norepinephrine inhibits it. So, although the net effect is an increase in brain activity, selegiline doesn't have a big effect as an instant aphrodisiac. That's why it is unlikely to become a drug of abuse, and has never gained favor as a street drug.

Selegiline works partly by blocking an enzyme called **monoamine oxidase (MAO),** that chews up dopamine. So it belongs to the well-known class of chemicals called MAO inhibitors, which includes many anti-depressants, such as phenelzine (Nardil), and tranylcypromine (Parnate).

MAO enzymes come in two types, MAO-A, mostly in your digestive system, and MAO-B, mostly in your brain. They both have essential functions. MAO-A has the important task of preventing build-up of the compound **tyramine** from your food. Tyramine will send your blood pressure over the moon. Many foods contain toxic levels of tyramine, including cheese, red wine, sardines, some beans, chocolate, and beer.

Over millions of years of evolution, Nature developed MAO-A to neutralize tyramine. If you block MAO-A, then you are asking for a hypertensive crisis. Medicine-men call it the "cheese reaction", because of the high levels of tyramine in gourmet cheeses. This deadly side-effect makes physicians very cautious about using MAO inhibitors.

But selegiline has a unique distinction that makes it a safe and effective component of the **Hormonal Health Program**. In moderate doses, selegiline inhibits only MAO-B enzymes in the brain. It leaves alone the MAO-A enzymes to do their vital work of breaking down tyramine in your gut.[4] At doses of 1-10 milligrams per day, which are effective for maintaining the brain dopamine system, selegiline is non-toxic. The **Physicians Desk Reference** notes that no cheese reactions have ever been reported with selegiline therapy.[2]

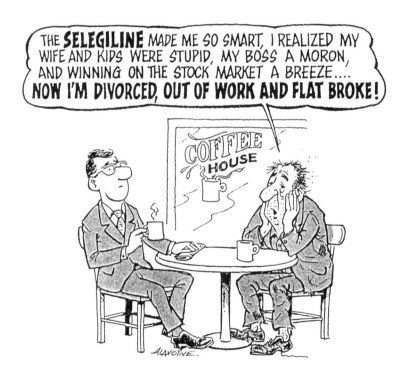

Dosage and Timing

Nevertheless, dosage is critical. Last year I was fielding questions on selegiline in the press tent at the Academy of Anti-Aging Medicine Convention, when a stentorian voice from the audience cut off the journalists. It came from an overweight man with a hard, red face like a book of rules. He complained, "I took up to 40 mg a day of deprenyl and all it did was make me sick." My reply, "I bet it drove your blood pressure way up, gave you headaches, and hurt your liver." "Sure did." He looked astonished. "No mystery. You were taking far too much. Forty milligrams a day will inhibit MAO-A as well as MAO-B. With your overweight and, I would guess, heavy job stress, and hypertension, that's asking for a stroke."

Selegiline is not innocuous. It's a powerful compound. Hypertension can occur with a dose of 20 milligrams.[5] Obviously, it should not be used at all by hypertensive folk, or folk taking other MAO inhibitors, or anti-depressants such as fluoxetine (Prozac) that interact with MAO inhibitors. As with every chemical discussed in this book, you should read the **Physicians Desk Reference** and get the advice of your physician before considering selegiline.

One of the inventors of selegiline, Dr. Joseph Knoll, Head of the Department of Pharmacology at Semmelweis University in Hungary, has been researching this chemical since 1960. He advocates only 1.0 - 2.0 milligrams per day to inhibit aging of the striatal dopamine system, rising to 5 milligrams per day three days a week, after age 60.[6] Treated with that proper respect, selegiline will improve the dopamine system in the striatal cortex in most people over age 30, and it will likely maintain it lifelong.

But it will not do well for folk who allow themselves to become fat, hypertensive, or overstressed. Selegiline is icing on the cake of a healthstyle life. It can't do much for you, unless you first reject the common Western lifestyle of junkfood-gobbling couch potatoism.

Hundreds of thousands of men and women throughout the world have been using tiny doses of selegiline for as much as 20 years, without harm, and with much apparent benefit. Members of the Colgan Institute have been using it since 1988. I must stress, however, that no controlled studies of selegiline have yet been done with healthy humans.

The best to date is a study of selegiline therapy with depressed men and women. Both sexes showed large improvements in confidence and well being, and also reported increased libido.[7] That sums up our experience too. With its known effects in maintaining striatal dopamine, selegiline forms an important part of the **Hormonal Health Program**.

Acetyl-L-Carnitine

To maintain your hormone cascade at youthful levels, you have to do everything possible to inhibit aging of the neurotransmitter systems of the striatal cortex and hypothalamus. One potent strategy is to increase the amount of the chemical **acetyl-L-carnitine** in your brain.

The natural amino acid L-carnitine occurs throughout your body and in many foods, including milk.[1] But you can't use simple L-carnitine supplements to maintain your brain. To get into the brain, supplements have to be in the *acetylated* form in order to pass easily through the blood-brain barrier. Once inside, acetyl-L-carnitine goes to work with a will.

I have space to cite only a couple of examples from the pile of more than 100 animal studies on my desk, showing that acetyl-L-carnitine protects the brain in multiple ways.[2-4] It is an antioxidant that prevents peroxidation of brain lipids.[5] That is, it prevents your brain, which is mostly made of fat, from going rancid. In turn this action reduces the build-up of **lipofuscin** (brown fats), cellular debris that interferes with brain function.[5] This non-toxic compound is so powerful, it even protects the optic nerves from aging.[4]

Protecting the visual system is particularly pertinent to humans, because failing vision is a prominent characteristic of usual human aging. No controlled studies have yet been done on normal humans to see if acetyl-L-carnitine will help. In diabetics, however, acetyl-L-carnitine is being used with some success to inhibit retinal damage common to this disease.[6]

In individual case studies at the Colgan Institute, we also have a number of reports of improved vision in folk who use acetyl-L-carnitine regularly. By improved, I mean that their optometrists have had to reduce the power of their glasses and contact lenses.

What have happy eyes to do with the hormone cascade? More than you think. The optic nerves wrap around and give off connections to the very areas of the hypothalamus that control your hormones. We have seen already, for example, how changes in visual stimulation control production of melatonin by the pineal gland, by visual signals to the suprachiasmatic nucleus of the hypothalamus. And you also learned in earlier chapters, how visual input can trigger libido by stimulating the hypothalamus. The intensity, colors, and shapes of the light hitting your eyes have multiple effects on your hormones.

The Acetylcholine Connection

From animal studies, we know that acetyl-L-carnitine supplements increase an enzyme called **acetylcoenzyme A**. This enzyme supports the acetylcholine system in the striatal cortex and hypothalamus, by providing material for another chemical, **carnitine-acetyltransferase,** that is essential to acetylcholine production.[7,8] Through this sequence, it's very likely that acetyl-L-carnitine supplements boost acetylcholine levels.

Healthy humans object to their brains being diced and sliced, so the human evidence is less direct. Nevertheless, carnitine-acetyltransferase is very low in the brains of folk who have died of Alzheimer's and other forms of senility.[9] And senility is closely linked with degeneration of the hippocampus in the striatal cortex. If acetyl-L-carnitine benefits acetylcholine metabolism in humans, it should help Alzheimer's as well as eyes.

It does. Multiple studies show large improvements in Alzheimers and other senile patients supplemented with acetyl-L-carnitine.[10,11] One of the most recent, was done by Dr. Jay Pettigrew and colleagues at the University of Pittsburgh Medical School. They found that Alzheimer's patients given acetyl-L-carnitine for a year showed far less mental deterioration than a control group. Measures of brain function using nuclear magnetic resonance, also showed less deterioration in the patients' brains than in the brains of controls.[10]

Effects are even more potent with mildly senile patients. A multi-center controlled trial in Italy, gave 500 patients a moderate supplement of 1500 mg of acetyl-L-carnitine per day for 90 days. Even in that short period, they showed significant improvements in intelligence, memory, and emotions. These effects persisted when tested again a month after supplementation ceased. Acetyl-L-carnitine will improve brain function even in brains that have been allowed to deteriorate beyond permanent repair. Taken before irreversible brain damage occurs, it can work wonders.

In a representative example, healthy men and women aged 22 - 27 were supplemented with moderate doses of acetyl-L-carnitine for 30 days. Complex video game tests before and after supplementation showed big improvements in speed of learning, speed of reaction, and reduction of errors, while on the acetyl-L-carnitine. This simple amino acid does more than just protect the brain, it can also improve normal cognition.[11]

Acetyl-L-Carnitine Boosts Dopamine

Because of its clear chemical connection to acetylcholine, not much research has been done yet, on effects of acetyl-L-carnitine on dopamine, the primary neurotransmitter that controls your hormone cascade. Animal studies now show that acetyl-L-carnitine benefits dopamine directly.[12]

Researchers at the Nathan Kline Institute in Orangeburg, New York, examined effects on dopamine release in the striatal cortex. They found that aged mice, given acetyl-L-carnitine for three months, showed much improved dopamine activity, despite an age-related loss of about half their dopamine receptors.[12]

The Kline Institute study was for only three months, and the aged animals used had already suffered a lot of irreversible cell death in their brains before it began. Studies using supplementation for longer periods, show that acetyl-L-carnitine can prevent much of the brain cell loss of usual aging if begun early enough. It inhibits cell loss not only in the striatal cortex, but also in the **prefrontal cortex,** your primary area for cognition, and in the **occipital cortex,** the brain area at the back of your head that is primary for vision.[13] If you start early, acetyl-L-carnitine may protect not only your hormone controls, but also other crutial parts of your brain.

Dosage and Timing

No one knows exactly how much acetyl-L-carnitine to use. Most studies have been done with doses of 500 - 2500 mg per day. At the Colgan Institute we use 1000 - 2000 mg, taken in the morning on rising. That's the best regime we know to synchronize the brain activity caused by acetyl-L-carnitine, with the rest of the hormone cascade.

Some researchers suggest taking acetyl-L-carnitine in the evening, because of the large release of hormones during sleep. Not a good idea. By stimulating the excitatory neurotransmitters acetylcholine and dopamine, acetyl-L-carnitine makes them dominant over the activity of the neurotransmitter **serotonin.** In your circadian rhythm, serotonin activity naturally becomes dominant at night and promotes sleep. Serotonin is also the base material from which your pineal gland makes melatonin. It's likely that acetyl-L-carnitine taken later than 3:00 - 4:00 p.m acts indirectly to suppress normal serotonin and melatonin activity, and disrupts both the hormone cascade and your sleep cycle.

No controlled trials have shown this action yet, but if you take a hearty dose of acetyl-L-carnitine at night, it should convince you in one try. After ten hours of itchy, twitchy insomnia, your morning mirror reveals eyes like holes burned in a blanket, over a mouth that mutters repeatedly, "Never, never, never again."

Used in the right way, however, acetyl-L-carnitine is a great boon to both brains and hormone cascades. But you have to begin while most of your brain cells are still alive and kicking. Don't delay. Take this book and the medical references to your physician right away.

The Coming Revolution

Right now the American Medical Association characterizes Alzheimers and various other forms of senility as diseases "with no effective treatment or prevention." And the usual treatment for failing hormones is an equally ineffective bolus of dangerous end-organ hormone. When the medicine men finally realize that prevention of brain degeneration, and protection of the hormone cascade, means starting in your 40's, the whole structure of health care will change utterly.

Acetyl-L-carnitine is the forerunner of many new neuroprotective compounds that can maintain your brain. In my forthcoming book, **Stop Aging,** I deal with a whole list of them including, **phosphatidylserine, centrophenoxine, linopiridine, vinpocetin** and **alpha-lipoic acid**. They provide such powerful protection that, within a decade, the evidence will force their acceptance into mainstream medicine. In the coming millenium, I predict that such anti-aging compounds will become as routine a part of health maintenance, as childhood inoculations and plugging the holes in your teeth.

─20

The DHEA Bandwagon

"New Hormone Stops Heart Disease." "Natural Hormone Extends Life." So played the headlines in 1986, after epidemiologist Elizabeth Barrett-Connor at the University of California, San Diego, published human data on **dehydroepiandrosterone (DHEA)**. She reported that men with *naturally* high levels of DHEA sulfate in their blood, suffered only half as many heart attacks as men with low DHEAS.[1] They also lived longer.

The media parade got it all wrong. DHEA is not new. It has been known and used for more than 50 years. Nor is there any evidence, that *artificially* raising **DHEA** levels by supplementation can extend human life.[2] Nevertheless, the apparent protection against heart disease, sparked a new academic focus on DHEA, across fields of research from anatomy to zoology.

By 1994, DHEA became world news. Roussel Uclaf, famous inventor of the French abortion pill RU486 (mifepristone), told paparazzi that DHEA is a "cure for aging."[3] That speculation hit thousands of newspapers as scientific truth, starting a public scramble for DHEA that has swelled to a stampede.

Such common confusion of speculation with evidence, illustrates two prevailing traits of Western civilization. First, many people still hold a medieval religious faith in miracles, especially when endorsed by a scientific authority. They vainly believe that the human condition can be cured by a magic pill.

Second, some scientists remain as arrogant as their Victorian forbears. They continue to believe that the ultimate problem posed by Nature, physical mortality, can be solved with a single chemical. Just because Uclaf and colleagues were smart enough to invent a high-tech way to **destroy** Nature's miracle of reproduction, they seem to think they're smart enough to **create**. Destruction is simple. Anyone can kill the mightiest tree with a handful of plastic explosive, but no one has yet created even a single living leaf.

DHEA: Just The Facts

Don't be misled: DHEA is no more a cure for aging than Ponce de Lyon's mythical fountain. It is only a small influence, just one of the many intermediate chemicals in your hormone cascade. Under the control of ACTH flowing from your pituitary, the cortex of your adrenal glands produces DHEA from cholesterol. Released into the blood as DHEA sulfate (DHEAS), it acts as an intermediate hormone, one function of which is to provide base material for manufacture of testosterone and estrogen.[2]

Though most of its other functions remain a mystery, thousands of scientists now believe the evidence strong enough to jump on the DHEA bandwagon. In June 1995, the New York Academy of Sciences hosted a three-day world conference on DHEA and aging. One of the speakers, leading biochemist Dr. Arthur Schwartz of Temple University School of Medicine, estimated that at least a quarter of the scientists there were using DHEA themselves.[4]

Distinguished oncologist and expert on the hormone, Dr. William Regelson at the Medical College of Virginia, admits he has been taking DHEA for five years.[4] He calls it the "Mother Steroid," and claims that, combined with melatonin, it could extend human life by up to 30 years.[4,5] Regelson walks his talk. Though chunky, in his seventies he looks 55, and is sharp as a tack.

Of Mice and Men

But single cases are not science: they give only tentative clues. The science of DHEA is almost all with rats and mice.[2,5] Feed these cow'rin' tim'rous beasties DHEA, and they show fat loss, reduced diabetes, reduced cardiovascular disease, reduced lung, breast, and other cancers, and improved intelligence.[2,4,6,7]

They also live longer.[4] The 1995 conference above, was awash with film of hoary old mice with rickety gait and falling hair, side-by-side with DHEA-supplemented mice of the same age, sporting shining coats and the scamper of youth.

Trouble is, mice are not men. Mice don't produce DHEA in their adrenals and have virtually none of the hormone. They are therefore likely to be much more sensitive to it. Small doses easily melt bodyfat in mice. But equivalent doses in humans have no effect. Even massive doses of 1.6 grams of DHEA per day failed to shift an ounce of blubber in studies of overweight men.[8,9]

The original heart-protection effect has also faded under the scrutiny of science. Dr. Elizabeth Barrett-Connor, who started the DHEA debacle in 1986, presented a large follow-up study in 1995, showing that men with high DHEA reduce their risk of heart disease by only 20%.[4] She wishes now she hadn't wasted a decade on it.

A "Buffer" Against Brain Aging

Despite these problems, DHEA still forms part of our **Hormonal Health Program**. Why? Because none of the human research to date has followed the basic principle of replacing other controllers upstream of DHEA in the hormone cascade, before replacing that particular hormone. Little wonder effects are disappointing.

Also, virtually none of the research has evaluated the individual differences in need for DHEA. Subjects with low blood DHEAS for their age, are likely to benefit far more than those with high blood DHEAS. When this research is done, I predict DHEA supplements will come out a winner.

I base this prediction on several grounds. First, DHEA is the most abundant steroid hormone in your body. Second, DHEA declines with usual aging more reliably than any other hormone. In men, DHEA declines in almost a straight line from your early twenties until death. In women the decline begins similarly, but shows a sharp drop with perimenopause (age 40-45). Thereafter, female DHEA declines in an almost straight line.[10,11] It is one of the most accurate predictors we know, of aging, disease, and death.[2,12]

Third, your brain contains many times more DHEA per gram of tissue than the rest of you. Animal research shows that DHEA in the brain, acts as a "buffer" against stress, which prevents brain cell damage.[13]

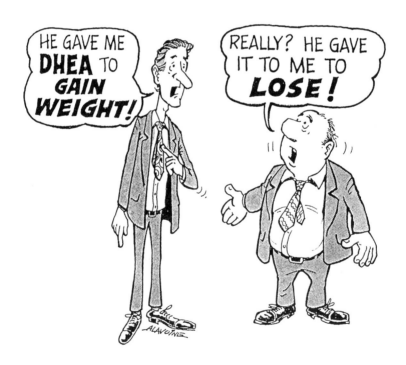

Human research also suggests it might protect our brains. In a study of senile men for example, 80% of those who required total nursing care had minuscule levels of DHEAS. Almost all the control group of normal men of similar ages showed higher DHEA levels.[14] Higher DHEA seems linked to the mental competence required to deal with everyday life.

Studies of Alzheimer's patients lend further support. DHEAS levels are much lower in folk with this disease than in controls of the same age.[15]

DHEA In The Hormone Cascade

Humans have such a complex hormone cascade, that DHEA plays different roles depending on the state of other hormones. In premenopausal women, for example, high levels of DHEAS are protective against breast cancer.[16] With the onset of perimenopause, however, DHEAS levels drop sharply.[17] After menopause, if estrogen is *not* replaced, then high DHEAS levels have the opposite effect, and *increase* the risk of breast cancer. DHEA seems to operate beneficially only in the presence of normal levels of other hormones.[18]

DHEA also seems to have only a small normal range at any particular age, so the window of beneficial supplementation may be very narrow. In mice, for example, low-dose DHEA enhances memory: high-dose DHEA inhibits memory.[19] That's why the **Hormonal Health Program** advocates using hormones in combination, from the brain down, and monitoring them regularly to ensure they all remain within youthful normal ranges.

DHEA Against Cancer

In women with normal estrogen levels, either natural or by hormone replacement, DHEA has a controlling effect on estrogen by binding some of its receptors.[20] That is, it stops excess estrogen from hooking onto these receptors and causing mischief.

Melatonin also binds estrogen receptors.[21] Replacing both melatonin and DHEA simultaneously to youthful levels, could well eliminate the risk of breast and reproductive cancers caused by estrogen replacement. So in the **Hormonal Health Program**, which always includes melatonin and estrogen replacement for postmenopausal women, DHEA supplementation adds vital protection against estrogen-induced cancers.

DHEA Protects Your Heart

Endocrinologist Dr. Peter Casson at Baylor College of Medicine, uses DHEA combined with estrogen for postmenopausal women. He reports improved immunity and a protective effect against cardiovascular disease.[22]

Given by itself, however, DHEA can *increase* cardiovascular risk in postmenopausal women, because it lowers HDL cholesterol.[23] But in women whose estrogen has been restored to within the normal range, DHEA increases cardiovascular protection.[24]

In men, DHEA is cardioprotective only in those with normal or high testosterone levels. In these men, who are usually slim, or at worst only a little overweight, DHEA appears to act as an estrogen, and reduces LDL cholesterol.[25]

Although they need help the most, DHEA will not protect badly overweight men from heart disease. These men are usually low in testosterone, and already too high in estrogen.[26] Bodyfat stores estrogen like crazy. They need to slim down first, before using replacement hormones.

These complex effects of DHEA underscore the need for the sort of multiple hormone replacement, nutrition, and exercise advocated by the **Hormonal Health Program**. If you are going to do hormone replacement at all, you have to do the whole enchilada.

DHEA Overdose

Most of the controlled trials of DHEA have used far too high a dose. DHEA at 1600mg per day for example, temporarily reduced bodyfat and increased muscle in normal weight men.[27] But you can bet your boots it was detrimental to other body functions.

When the same 1600mg dose was given to postmenopausal women, after two weeks their DHEAS levels jumped 20-fold. These extreme levels of DHEA went completely out-of-control, and transformed into high levels of both androgens and estrogens. Testosterone levels, for example, jumped 9-fold.[28]

There is no way your body can operate properly with uncontrollable levels of hormones, whizzing around the bloodstream looking for trouble.

The **Hormonal Health Program** focuses on restoring hormones only to their normal youthful ranges. These are the only levels known to science that are consistent with health and vitality. Anyone who tells you they are taking high doses of DHEA, and getting younger, slimmer, healthier, or smarter, watch them. A year or so later, they'll be older, fatter, sicker, and dumber.

DHEA: The Right Way

It doesn't take much DHEA to restore body levels, even in older folk. The new work of Dr. Arlene Morales and colleagues at the University of California, San Diego provides a representative example.[29] They gave men and women aged 40 - 70, a reasonable dose of 50mg of oral DHEA per day for three months. Blood levels of DHEA and DHEAS were quickly restored to those of normal 20-year-olds, and stayed there. Estrogen levels remained unchanged in both sexes. Testosterone increased only in women, and then only within the normal female range.

Levels of one other hormone did increase, **insulin-like growth factor 1 (IGF-1)**, but again only within the normal range. As you will see in the chapter on growth hormone, IGF-1 maintains muscle mass and inhibits fat gain. IGF-1 also declines with aging. So this effect of DHEA, like its mild boost of testosterone in women, probably represents beneficial physiological adjustments of the hormone cascade to a more youthful pattern.

DHEA Boosts Mood, Muscle, and Immunity

Other findings by Morales support the biochemical evidence. Almost all her subjects, both male and female showed substantial improvements in physical and psychological well-being.

The research of Morales' colleague, Dr. Samuel Yen at the University of California, San Diego, offers further support. Since 1991 he has given men and women just enough DHEA to replace their age-related losses. His supplementation periods of 3-6 months are still too short, but liability concerns naturally limit all human research into the unknown. Despite the limitation, Yen reports increased well-being, improved immune function, and increased muscle mass.[22]

For the past four years, the Colgan Institute has been following individuals who have chosen to use similar, small replacement doses of DHEA continuously. We have found that the benefits to well-being, physique, and resistance to disease have continued throughout the whole period.

The Insulin Connection

Under the prediabetic condition of insulin resistance, insulin loses its ability to deal with blood sugar. Blood sugar gradually rises to dangerous levels. Responding to signals of excess blood sugar, the pancreas gland pumps out more and more insulin. After a few years, both blood sugar and blood insulin become too high for health.

The liver responds to the dangerous levels of both insulin and sugar by frantically converting them to less poisonous fat. But the syndrome continues. In a decade or so, you have a typical overweight 50-year-old, who cannot lose much weight by dieting, and who has blood full of insulin, sugar, and fat.[30] These are the walking timebombs who explode into fatal heart attacks every day in the streets and boardrooms of modern America.

We saw in previous chapters how normal estrogen levels help to protect women from insulin resistance. But estrogen by itself is insufficient. Some premenopausal women have plenty of estrogen, but still develop insulin resistance. New studies show that these women have low levels of DHEAS.[31]

The decline of testosterone in males with usual aging, is also linked to DHEA and insulin resistance. Men with low testosterone, also typically have low DHEAS levels. Recent studies show a strong link between low levels of both hormones, and the high blood insulin and high blood sugar of insulin resistance.[32]

In strains of mice prone to insulin resistance and diabetes, DHEA stops the disease stone dead.[33] It also dramatically improves insulin sensitivity in normal mice.[34]

Research in humans has only just begun, but confirms the animal work. A new study on postmenopausal women, shows that 50mg of DHEA per day enhances insulin sensitivity and lowers blood triglycerides (fats).[35] Future human research is likely to show that DHEA supplementation can help prevent America's current epidemic of insulin resistance, and its accompanying obesity, diabetes, and cardiovascular risk.

In postmenopausal women, it's likely that the combination of hormones proposed by the **Hormonal Health Program** will yield even more dramatic results. These include melatonin to synchronize the hormone cascade and control estrogen, DHEA to prevent insulin resistance and fat deposition, and also to control estrogen, and estrogen itself for its prevention of insulin resistance, and its multiple other benefits. I predict that these strategies will produce a new breed of older women, never before seen on this Earth, smarter, happier, slimmer, more beautiful, and highly resistant to disease.

Dose and Timing

Though not an approved drug in America, thousands of physicians now prescribe DHEA like candy, for myriad aging ailments, from erectile dysfunction in men, to breast cancer in women, and overweight and Alzheimer's disease in anyone. The drug is readily available from compounding pharmacies, some mail order companies, and, very cheaply, from AIDS hotlines. Folk with AIDS have used DHEA in huge doses for over a decade, but without success. Overdosing DHEA hasn't done much good for other diseases either.

Fat-busting is a good example. Large doses of DHEA have no long-term effect in reducing bodyfat, and the small doses sufficient for replacement, *taken without other hormones*, simply shift fat from the thighs and hips to the belly. Studies confirming our findings with individual cases, show that this fat transfer occurs both in men and in premenopausal and postmenopausal women.[35-37]

The **Hormonal Health Program** recommends no more than 25-50mg of DHEA per day. We take it for only five days per week, as a crude strategy to prevent possible feedback suppression of natural hormone production. Recent evidence suggests that DHEA interacts in complex ways with dopamine in the hypothalamus, so continuous use might cause negative feedback suppression of brain hormones.[38]

Because of reported stimulation of energy by DHEA, we take it only in the morning, so as to avoid possible sleep disturbance. No one knows the right time to take DHEA, but the natural circadian burst of testosterone in mid-morning,[39] suggests it may be least disruptive to testosterone rhythms if taken on rising.

We get DHEAS measured every 3-6 months, and adjust replacement dosages to keep blood levels no higher than the mid-normal range for a 25-year-old. DHEAS ranges for adults (20-25) are:

Males:	2800-4000 ng/ml
Females:	1600-3000 ng/ml

Physicians can order reliable DHEAS tests from Metpath Laboratories at 800-631-1390.

Before you rush off to get DHEA, first take this book and the medical references to your physician. If you do decide to use it, you do so at your own choice and risk. Remember, the research I have reviewed is on the cutting edge of hormone replacement. As yet, DHEA has no long-term controlled trials on humans to recommend it.

21

Growth Hormone

On the 5th of July, 1990, Dr. Daniel Rudman and an army of researchers at the Medical College of Wisconsin and Chicago University Medical School, reported that injections of growth hormone *reversed* some degenerative changes of aging in old men.

Twelve men aged 61-81, who showed low levels of **insulin-like growth factor-1 (IGF-1)**, were given injections of synthetic human growth hormone three times a week for six months. Doses were varied so as to raise their IGF-1 to the middle of the youthful range and keep it there. A matched control group got dummy injections. The study was impeccably designed and conducted. After six months on growth hormone, the men showed a 9% increase in lean mass, a 14% decrease in bodyfat, a 1.6% increase in bone density, and a 7% increase in skin thickness. The controls showed none of these benefits.[1]

Media reports inflated these modest findings into a "reversal of 10 - 20 years of aging", and sparked a demand for growth hormone by older Americans, that is making the manufacturers as rich as Croesus.[2] Rudman's experimental test of the drug was exemplary and innovative research. But medical use of it in the same way is such an obvious error, I have to conclude, that the greed of the physicians involved is matched only by their stupidity.

Growth Hormone: Basics

To understand this stupidity, requires only basic knowledge of growth hormone. It forms part of the hormone cascade from your pituitary gland every day of your life. Most of it is released at night. But a variety of other conditions, including exercise and food deprivation, also cause growth hormone release.

Young men make 0.4 - 1.0 mg per day, young women a little more. That level of production maintains a store of 5 - 10 mg in your pituitary. Without it you would die.[3]

Growth hormone is released in bursts, which travel in your bloodstream to the liver, where almost all of it is destroyed within an hour. So despite its name, growth hormone can't cause growth directly.

The process of growth hormone destruction by your liver, produces other chemicals called **insulin-like growth factors (IGFs).** The one we know most about is dubbed, **IGF-1.** In combination with insulin, IGF-1 travels to the muscles, tendons and ligaments, where it maintains growth of lean tissue. It also travels to the adipose cells, where it again interacts with insulin to promote release of bodyfat into the blood for use as fuel.[4]

Because growth hormone comes in bursts and is quickly destroyed, blood levels are almost impossible to measure accurately. IGF-1 levels, however, are reasonably stable. Now you understand why Rudman and other researchers measure IGF-1 to estimate a subject's need for growth hormone.

Does Growth Hormone Decline With Aging?

Measurements of representative samples of Western populations, show that growth hormone levels and IGF-1 levels decline with usual aging.[5,6] But as I've pointed out earlier in this book, to be representative, samples of the public have to contain many subjects who are overweight and sedentary. Despite the error of inferring normal human functions from such folk, it is still common medical belief that declining growth hormone is an inevitable consequence of the passing years.

Let's examine the facts. First, measurement of 24-hour growth hormone fails to detect any of the hormone in some healthy young folk. Second, some subjects with very low levels of growth hormone, have higher levels of IGF-1 than subjects with normal levels of growth hormone.[7,8] So growth hormone level is not as closely linked with IGF-1 as clinicians would like to think.

Third, many healthy older people have higher levels of growth hormone *and* IGF-1 than healthy young people.[9] So growth hormone and IGF-1 levels do not necessarily decline with aging.

Fourth, growth hormone and IGF-1 levels are profoundly affected by exercise. Sedentary subjects have much lower levels than subjects who exercise regularly, no matter how old they are. Some studies report that IGF-1 is related more to VO_2 max, and other measures of physical fitness, than to age.[10]

You can't justify a need for growth hormone by its effects either. When you give growth hormone to young men, who already show ample growth hormone of their own, it has exactly the same effects on body composition as in old men who have low growth hormone. They lose bodyfat and gain muscle.[11] If growth hormone causes the same changes in both young and old, whether or not they are deficient, its effects can hardly be called "rejuvenation."

Dangers of Growth Hormone

Nevertheless, medical use of growth hormone "replacement therapy" is growing at a wild pace. American and European clinics are citing Rudman's work as "reversal of aging", and offering the same therapy for anyone in full page ads in national magazines.[12] It's the health care of the century.

Experimental research with growth hormone has to be much more precise than clinical use of the drug. Researchers use stringent criteria and repeated multiple measurements to define their subjects. They have to tread their way through the maze of measurement uncertainties, so as to select only those people with a true growth hormone deficiency. Otherwise their results disappear like smoke in the statistical analysis, and the work never gets published.

Clinicians, however, often give growth hormone after only perfunctory testing.   We have numerous reports at the Colgan Institute, of growth hormone being prescribed after only a patient interview and a minimal physical exam, especially by Mexican clinics.

Crazy!   Growth hormone is not candy.   It's the most powerful anabolic hormone known to science. Even with the best of experimental controls to define those that need it, and then to keep their growth hormone levels within the normal range, it has repeatedly proved toxic.

More than half of Rudman's patients dropped out within a year because of side-effects. Rudman himself died, but other researchers who were initially enthusiastic about the drug, are now back-peddling furiously.

Drs. Kevin Yarasheski and Jeffrey Zachwieja of Washington University School of Medicine used only low doses of growth hormone in very carefully screened subjects 63 - 76 years of age. In both men and women, these physiological doses of growth hormone caused a high incidence of carpal tunnel syndrome, fluid retention, and arthralgia (joint pain). After all this discomfort they found, "Growth hormone recipients who completed four months of treatment have *not* exhibited extraordinary improvements in body composition." (Italiacs mine). No wonder they entitled their report, "The Fountain of Youth Proves Toxic."[13]

Pancreas Problems

Growth hormone also whacks your pancreas gland. The clues were there, both in the known functions of growth hormone and in the results of Rudman's study. But the researchers were so set on proving rejuvenation, they missed the evidence staring them in the face.

The biochemistry of your hormone cascade is precise. In order to work, growth hormone requires insulin. If you put in extra growth hormone, you put a demand on the body to produce extra insulin. But researchers gave no support to the aging pancreas glands of their patients. The inevitable result was enormous stress on the pancreas to produce more insulin, and its gradual decline from overwork.

Rudman's results showed increased blood sugar levels in patients on growth hormone.[1] Other reports showed hyper-secretion of insulin.[14] No surprise then, that subjects frequently have to drop out of growth hormone studies, or have to stop clinically prescribed growth hormone, because they develop pancreatitis, hyperglycemia (high blood sugar), insulin resistance, or full-blown adult-onset diabetes[15-18] It's not worth risking the curse of diabetes for a little more muscle and energy. There are far better ways to increase your growth hormone and IGF-1 than by shooting it up.

Alternatives to Growth Hormone

I have already noted above how exercise can increase growth hormone and IGF-1. You will see precisely how to do it in the exercise chapter ahead. And, as I show in the nutrition chapter, specific supplements can also do the trick, with no toxicity or side-effects. But there's one other chemical in the hormone cascade that raises IGF-1 nicely - DHEA.

The best subjects to demonstrate this effect are postmenopausal woman. At perimenopause and thereafter, DHEA levels drop sharply. Supplemental DHEA increases not only testosterone in these women, but also IGF-1.[19]

There is a place for growth hormone in the **Hormonal Health Program**, but only for folk who have a precisely defined growth hormone deficiency, tested and verified repeatedly by a good endocrinologist. Even then, growth hormone should be used only after the whole hormone cascade has been supported for at least six months by your physician, and you have followed the nutrition and exercise program. If growth hormone remains low, which is unlikely, only then should you consider using it. Otherwise, all that you get for the princely sum of $15,000 per year, is a particularly poisonous pig in a poke.

22

Testosterone For Men

In a 1992 article, "Futures in Testosterone," I recommended that investors forget about pork bellies, and pin their financial hopes on male hormones. The market has proved it. Testosterone sales have jumped by the hundreds of millions of $$$, fueled by reports of rejuvenation and vitality.

Some examples: Dr. Eric Orwell, of Oregon Health Sciences University, states that men aged 60-75, showed improved spatial intelligence when they wore scrotal testosterone patches."[1] **The Wall Street Journal** reports that testosterone patches improve libido, emotions and sexual performance.[2] Dr. Rahmawhati Sih of St. Louis University Medical School reports, that twice weekly testosterone injections made men stronger, gave them larger muscles, and lowered their cholesterol. As for sex, Dr. Sih (a woman) comments, "Their wives really knew it."[3]

In Europe new clinics that treat "viripause" (male menopause) with testosterone are doing brisk trade. In America testosterone sales have tripled since 1987. What's happening here? How did a hormone that's been used in medicine for 60 years,[4] suddenly become the new nirvana?

Testosterone Declines With Usual Aging

What's happening is research over the last two decades, suggesting that men decline into feeble frailty, not because of inevitable aging, but rather because of low testosterone levels.

We saw in Chapter 1 how male impotence in America has doubled since the 1940s. The average modern man is a wimp compared with his forefathers. With a mass of aging baby-boomers swelling the low testosterone ranks, the quest to remain as virile as Sean Connery, Robert Redford or Jack Nicholson grows more urgent by the day.

At least 15 studies and reviews between 1970 and 1995, report declines in male testosterone levels with usual aging.[5] Numerous researchers have wrongly assumed this decline to be primary degeneration of the testes, which permanently reduces their ability to manufacture the hormone. Physicians have jumped in with pills, shots, and patches of testosterone to restore its status. The immediate result for aging males is physical and mental virility. As we will see, the long-term result is health disaster.

Only now, in the late 1990s, are scientists asking the right questions. What changes in the hormone cascade reduce testosterone? What other factors interfere with testosterone production? And what interventions can we make to restore testosterone, without resorting to the dangerous end-organ hormone itself?

Navigating the Testosterone Cascade

Right at the top of the cascade, new studies show that the decline of pineal melatonin with aging, is linked to reduced pituitary production of **adrenocorticotrophic hormone (ACTH)**.[6] ACTH is primary for conversion of cholesterol to pregnenolone and DHEA at the adrenals, the base materials for testosterone and all other steroid hormones. When ACTH levels fall, so do testosterone levels. Melatonin is clearly one hormone that should be restored before considering testosterone.

The adrenal hormone **dehydroepiandrosterone (DHEA)** itself declines with aging, probably because of a decline in enzyme function at the adrenals.[7-9] DHEA supplementation is a second option to explore before contemplating testosterone.

Other studies report a decline with aging in the pituitary hormone, **luteinizing hormone**, which controls manufacture of testosterone by the testes.[10,11] Since release of luteinizing hormone is stimulated by activity of the neurotransmitter **dopamine** in the hypothalamus, this evidence indicates probable degeneration of dopamine function.

Evidence also shows that pituitary manufacture of prolactin tends to rise with age. That's a strong sign of degeneration of hypothalamic dopamine, because prolactin output is kept down by *inhibitory* action of dopamine. When dopamine function declines with usual aging, it reduces the whole hormone cascade, including testosterone.[12] Restoration of dopamine function with **selegiline** should always be tried before resorting to testosterone.

Dopamine works hand-in-hand with the neurotransmitter **acetylcholine**. Because acetylcholine function also declines with aging, restoration with **acetyl-l-carnitine** may be crucial. Especially so when you consider the rapidly rising incidence of Alzheimer's disease, which is strongly linked to acetylcholine decline and brain cell death in the striatal cortex.

Nutrition Affects Testosterone

Nutritional deficiencies also cause testosterone decline. Space prevents me covering all the deficiencies involved, so I will use **zinc** as a pertinent example. The majority of older men show low zinc intake and poor zinc nutritional status.[4] Zinc deficiency is a well established cause of testicular degeneration and testosterone decline.[13,14]

Unlike testosterone, zinc supplementation is completely non-toxic, has no detrimental side-effects, and can often cure the problem. Other nutritional strategies that affect testosterone and sexual potency are covered in the nutrition chapter ahead.

Medication Whacks Testosterone

You saw in Chapter 8 the huge number of prescription drugs that produce impotence as a side-effect. Drugs that interfere with the hormone cascade include, anti-hypertensives, diuretics, anti-depressants, tranquilizers, and thyroid hormones.

If you are on any of these medications (see Tables in Chapter 8), then testosterone injections or patches will likely worsen the disease you are being treated for. Rather than mess with male hormones, ask your physician, and study the **Physician's Desk Reference**, for alternative medication that doesn't have wimp as a prominent side-effect.

Testosterone: Not A Primary Deficiency

As you can see, the multiple causes of testosterone decline, show it is rarely a problem of the testes alone. Consequently, meddling with this end-organ hormone, without first attending to other causes of low testosterone, is a big mistake. The current rash of ad lib testosterone replacement, which attempts to correct general debility or sexual dysfunction in aging baby-boomers, is yet another sick joke of American health care.

Testosterone therapy, especially given alone, for any purpose but *documented* testicular degeneration, simply adds to the deficits upstream in the hormone cascade. Within a few months, the excess testosterone levels in the blood send negative feedback to the hypothalamus, which further reduces function throughout the cascade.[15] Exogenous testosterone is so good at shutting down the hypothalamus and pituitary, it is being tested as a male contraceptive by the World Health Organization.[16]

Instead of testosterone, the **Hormonal Health Program** advocates judicious use of melatonin to compensate for pineal deficits,[17] selegiline and acetyl-l-carnitine to improve dopamine and acetylcholine function in the hypothalamus,[18] DHEA to increase available substrate for testosterone,[19] removal of offending medications, and a full spectrum vitamin, mineral, and antioxidant supplement and nutrition program,[20] to correct nutritional deficiencies. These strategies provide a virtually non-toxic, alternative to testosterone therapy, with negligible side-effects and numerous long-term benefits.

When Testosterone is Required

About 10% of men age 40-60 and 20% aged 60-80 do show some evidence of testicular degeneration.[21] These folk do require testosterone replacement in addition to the above strategies, just as women require estrogen replacement for primary ovarian decline. The usual testosterones, however, cause more problems than they alleviate.

To understand these problems, first you have to realize that testosterone is an anabolic steroid. Why then is it being prescribed freely, when other anabolic steroids are considered as illegal as narcotics? They are all tightly controlled by the Drug Enforcement Administration (DEA) under the Anabolic Steroids Control Act of 1990. For even possessing these drugs, you are likely to lose your house, your car, and your children, and spend the rest of your life marked as a criminal.

The answer is, neither the DEA nor the Food and Drug Administration (FDA) dare touch testosterone, even though it is also listed under the Act. Too many influential folk are using it, including aging senators, congressmen, state attorneys and senior policemen. The frisky, aging lawmaker or law enforcer, would object mightily if he was accused of using anabolic steroids. But that is exactly what they are doing.

The irony of this whole situation, is that the banned forms of anabolic steroids were developed precisely so as to be more effective and safer than testosterone. Yet the very aging yuppies who now clamor for male hormones, are the same folk who clamored for them to be banned in the '80s, because of abuse by athletes and teenagers. By ignorant lawmaking, the folk who now need the safe forms of testosterone the most, have put them beyond their own reach.

For the usual testosterone replacement therapy, they are stuck with the old anabolic steroids, **methyltestosterone**, **testosterone propionate**, and **testosterone enanthate**.

Methyltestosterone

Methyltestosterone is an anabolic steroid created 40 years ago, the first form that could be taken orally. It is also one of the most toxic and ineffective forms.

Like the newer, safer, and more effective orals, **methandrostenolone** (Dianabol) and **oxandrolone** (Anavar), methyltestosterone is simply synthetic testosterone chemically altered to reduce its destruction by the liver. The obsolete chemistry still used to produce methyltestosterone, is not a good fit to the human body. Long-term use can produce a plethora of disorders including, depression, liver inflammation, liver cysts, and liver cancer.[22,23]

Benefits from the usual prescription of methyltestosterone are doubtful anyway. It comes in 10mg and 25mg tablets, which prescription records show, has led many physicians to believe that 25 - 50 mg represents an effective daily dose. The **Physician's Desk Reference**, however, states that,

> doses as high as 400 mg per day are needed to achieve clinically effective blood levels for full replacement therapy[24]

At such a dose, liver disorders and other side-effects are highly likely. Especially so, because methyltestosterone is prescribed without any effective strategy, to time the induced rise in blood testosterone, so that it is in synchrony with the 24-hour rhythm of the hormone cascade.

Testosterone Propionate and Enanthate

Injection of testosterone fires a big bolus of the drug into your body, which would send blood levels into the stratosphere. To overcome this problem, the **propionate** and **enanthate** forms of testosterone are chemically altered to remove their water, thus making them more fat-soluble. Consequently, when injected, some of the testosterone is held in your body fats and, hopefully, only slowly released into the blood as free testosterone.

Despite these hopes, the weekly or twice weekly injections of 50-200mg of these drugs, produce a pattern of testosterone highs and lows that bears no relation to the hormone cascade. Immediately after injection blood testosterone levels rise precipitously. By the time for the next injection, levels fall to below normal.

Over the past decade, the Colgan Institute has provided information to hundreds of physicians and patients, who have experienced problems with long-term use of injectable testosterones. These problems include prostate enlargement, depression, and impotence. Indeed, the World Health Organization reports, that one 200mg injection of testosterone enanthate per week is an effective male contraceptive.[25]

For hormone replacement, testosterone injections are little advanced on the shenanigans of French physician Dr. Brown-Sequard, who started it all back in 1889. He sought rejuvenation by injecting himself with extracts made from the testicles of freshly killed dogs.[26] Though he noisily proclaimed success, after a couple of years Brown-Sequard degenerated miserably. Anyone today who uses the comparable strategy of testosterone injections, will likely suffer the same fate.[27]

The Patch

Testosterone delivery through the skin is the only way to go. After interminable delays, the technology developed for transdermal delivery of scopolamine to prevent motion sickness, and nitroglycerin to prevent heart attacks, is now delivering hormones too. For the first time in history, we have a system capable of mimicking your natural testosterone output.

First came the **Testoderm** scrotal patch, developed by Alza Pharmaceuticals in Palo Alto, California, and approved by the FDA in October 1993. A three-inch square patch is lightly stuck on the shaved scrotum, worn for 22 hours, and replaced with a new one. The patch, contains a gel film impregnated with either 4mg or 6mg of pure testosterone. Correct use will raise blood testosterone into the normal range in almost all men with testicular deficits of the hormone.[28,29]

The most important benefit created by the patch, is delivery of testosterone to your body in synchrony with your hormone cascade. The normal circadian rhythm of testosterone, involves a mid-morning peak and a gradual decline until night.[30] Applying the Testoderm patch in the early morning, allows induced blood levels to mimic this pattern, and thus be synchronized with the rhythm of natural testosterone output.

Obsolete oral and injectable testosterone therapies have to use toxic doses of hundreds of milligrams in order to achieve an effect. The Testoderm patch comes in 4mg and 6mg, which approximates the range of daily testosterone output in young men (5mg-7mg), and achieves a superior effect. With these physiological doses, the Testoderm patch achieves levels of testosterone that plateau within the normal range after about four weeks.[31]

So, using the patch, you get none of the peaks and valleys of testosterone that cause much of the trouble with older therapies. Also, without excess blood testosterone to send negative feedback to the hypothalamus, suppression of the hormone cascade is unlikely.

The only disadvantage of Testoderm use, is a rise in **dihydrotestosterone** levels to three times the normal average. This effect seems to occur by conversion of testosterone to dihydrotestosterone, by the high levels of the enzyme **5-alpha-reductase** in scrotal skin. Excess dihydrotestosterone is linked to overgrowth of the prostate, though no such overgrowth is reported with Testoderm therapy. If you do use it though, read the chapter herein on prostate problems. The non-toxic European remedy, pygeum/saw palmetto, effectively suppresses conversion of testosterone to dihydrotestosterone.

The Androderm Patch

The latest development is the **Androderm** patch, developed by TheraTech in Salt Lake City, Utah. Licensed by SmithKline Beecham, Androderm was approved by the FDA on 2 October 1995. The advantage of Androderm is, it can be stuck on the back, belly, thighs or upper arms.

Two Androderms deliver a physiological dose of 5mg of pure testosterone per day. So early morning application should mimic the normal rhythm and level of testosterone in the hormone cascade. Absorption with this patch may be slower than with Testoderm, however, because the manufacturers recommend application at night.

Back, belly, thigh, and arm skin do not have a lot of the 5-alpha-reductase enzyme. So Androderm patches do not raise dihydrotestosterone to excessive levels. This advantage, plus the flexibility to use one, two, or three patches to achieve normal testosterone levels, gives Androderm my nod as the best method yet for testosterone replacement.

23

Testosterone For Women

Even Tim Allen's ape grunt can't save the myth of male testosterone dominance. Earlier chapters showed you how testosterone is also a female hormone, firing libido, well-being, confidence, leadership, and zest for life equally in both men and women.

Physicians I know, still believe what they were taught in medical school. About 40% of a woman's testosterone is manufactured in her ovaries. Most of the rest is manufactured in her adrenal glands, and both sources of testosterone production continue unchanged after menopause. So women don't need testosterone replacement. These beliefs are false.

Nevertheless, they set the course for hormone replacement. When estrogen first became available in the early '60s, American and British medical authorities discouraged the addition of testosterone. They continued to do so for the next 30 years, thereby condemning hundreds of millions of postmenopausal women to emotional and sexual disorder.

All the additional millions of women who lost their ovaries to hysterectomy, were dismissed with an airy wave of the chauvinist hand, as being able to cope with the testosterone provided by their adrenals. These women suffer the worst because, without ovaries, the testosterone profile is grim indeed. To protect you from a similar fate, here is the real science of female testosterone.

The Female Testosterone System

Contrary to many medical texts, neither the ovaries nor the adrenals are the main source of a woman's testosterone. The recent research of Dr. Christopher Longcope, at the University of Massachusetts Medical School, and other scientists, has shown conclusively that the skin, muscles, bodyfat, and brain of young women, manufacture more testosterone than their ovaries and adrenals combined.[1] They produce this miracle by conversion of steroid intermediates, mainly our old friend dehydroepiandrosterone (DHEA).

Average ovarian production of testosterone is about 50 micrograms per day. Average adrenal production is also about 50 micrograms per day. Average production from other tissues is 100 - 150 micrograms per day.[2] That yields a total of 200 - 250 micrograms of testosterone per day in healthy young women. That's the average amount they need for sexual and emotional potency.

At perimenopause (age 40 - 45) everything changes. Ovarian production of testosterone slows down, but not by a lot.[1,3] This minor decline in what used to be considered the main source of female testosterone, spawned the false medical belief that adequate female testosterone levels continue after menopause.

Not a chance. Blood testosterone falls through the floor at perimenopause, because adrenal and other organ production declines drastically. Adrenal testosterone falls by 40 - 50%. Testosterone from skin, muscles, bodyfat, and brain, the main source of the hormone in women, falls by 60% or more.[4] That leaves a total of about 50 - 100 micrograms of testosterone in menopausal women, less than half their normal supply.

Women who lose their ovaries to surgery fare worst, because they lose an additional 40 - 50 micrograms per day. There is no way that libido, energy, confidence, well-being, joy or passion can function properly under such a restriction.

A representative case that gained media attention was Dr. Anita Sacks, a prominent psychoanalyst who had a hysterectomy at age 46. For two years afterwards she took estrogen replacement, but never felt her usual self. In her own words,

> I was lacking more than my
> libido -- my life force was gone.

Dr. Sacks trudged the usual medical road for years before she found a physician who knew what he was doing. She was prescribed **Estratest** (combined estrogen and methyltestosterone).

Even though this is a crude drug, after a year or so she returned to full vitality.

Testosterone Replacement

Dr. Barbara Sherwin has been reporting similar benefits from testosterone in repeated controlled studies since the early 80's. Hysterectomized women only recover their full energy and well being when testosterone is added to estrogen replacement[5,6]. She has also shown repeatedly that postmenopausal women given testosterone, develop higher energy, more zest and more positive emotions.[7]

Though studies of testosterone replacement in *clinically* depressed women have yet to be done, subjects in the research of Sherwin and others, show dramatic relief from depressive symptoms.[7,8] Because the line between clinical depression and everyday depression is often defined by the scrawl of a physician's signature on a prescription for antidepressants, in many cases a little testosterone may be all that is required. Even after 20 years of evidence, however, testosterone is still not approved for treatment of post-menopausal depression, because of the prevailing myth that women don't need it - period.

After reading the research I gave him, one of my ob/gyn colleagues expressed the common medical attitude. He acknowledged the findings but still refused to give women testosterone. His reasoning:

> They don't need it. Libidinous 50-year-
> olds would be bad enough, but I would
> hate to have my patients, or the women

who run this hospital suddenly turn aggressive.

The covert desire of medicine men to keep postmenopausal women docile and compliant, may have been more of an influence on replacement therapy than they want you to know.

No Heart Problems

Another medical reason advanced for not allowing women testosterone, is the notion that it would cancel out the cardiovascular protection afforded by estrogen replacement. Women who have high testosterone levels show lower levels of protective HDL cholesterol, and higher levels of damaging LDL cholesterol, so have a higher risk of heart disease.[9] This reasoning, however, confuses excessive testosterone with testosterone restored to normal youthful levels. For the truth, let's go to the evidence.

Research with monkeys, indicates that hearts do just fine with a modicum of the big T. Dr. Janice Wagner and colleagues at Bowman Gray School of Medicine in Winston Salem, North Carolina, gave postmenopausal macaques either estrogen or estrogen plus testosterone replacement. Both groups showed exactly the same degree of protection against cardiovascular degeneration.[10] A control group given no hormone replacement, degenerated rapidly.

Research with women agrees. Dr. Barbara Sherwin and colleagues for example, compared groups of women who had suffered full hysterectomy four years previously. One group had been on estrogen replacement, the second on estrogen plus testosterone. The third group had opted not to take hormones. The three groups showed no difference in HDL, LDL or serum cholesterol levels.[11] Other studies confirm Sherwin's findings that a modicum of testosterone does not reduce a woman's protection against cardiovascular disease.[12]

Testosterone May Protect Against Lupus

Testosterone may even be protective against another degenerative disease suffered predominantly by women - **lupus erythymatosis**. New research suggests that lupus is caused primarily by the high levels of estrogen in women. Estrogen boosts the female immune system to such a degree, that eventually it begins to attack the body itself. Very few men get lupus, because their testosterone protects them by damping estrogen's effects.[13]

The new evidence of testosterone as an estrogen controller, is only just entering the medical literature. As it is progressively adopted into practice, we will see a big change in the medical attitude to testosterone for women. Estrogen *without* testosterone will then be cast in its proper light - an incomplete and dangerous form of hormone replacement.

Forms of Testosterone

The 30-year neglect of postmenopausal women's need for testosterone, is nowhere better illustrated than in the history of the drug itself. Now that the gig is up and women everywhere are demanding testosterone, medicine men are making a big play of providing it.

Estratest (estrogen plus methyltestosterone) is being lauded by the media as a new advance. Even some physicians think it's a recent drug. **Premarin with methyltestosterone** is also getting good press. The general impression given, is that medicine is doing its bit to provide better medication in line with recent evidence of women's needs.

What a laugh! When I first became interested in hormone replacement in 1981, both Estratest and Premarin with methytestosterone were already approved and already in the **Physicians Desk Reference**, with the identical formulations now shown in the **1996 Physicians Desk Reference.**[14,15] In fact, Estratest was approved in 1965, over 30 years ago.[16] There's nothing new about them at all.

These drugs languished for three decades because most physicians would not prescribe them. The evidence was clear and unequivocal by the early '80s. I leave it to you gentle reader, to judge the motivation behind their failure to provide the approved health care.

Obsolete Drugs

The above two forms of combined estrogen and testosterone replacement are still the only two approved for women. They may have been state of the art in the '60s, but now they are way out of date. As I reviewed in the Testosterone for Men chapter, methyltestosterone is one of the least effective and most toxic anabolic steroids. Both replacement drugs available for women in America still contain only methyltestosterone.

Meanwhile, patch technology for men uses pure testosterone, a much safer and more effective hormone. No testosterone patches are yet available for women. No testosterone cream is yet approved, implants are abysmal, and sublingual testosterone is still on the drawing board.

The irony is that the majority of women need a smidgen of testosterone from perimenopause on, and for the 30 - 40 years of life thereafter. But only a minority of men *ever* need testosterone, and most of those only in their last decade. Yet they are getting all the attention. High time we prodded the political parade to get their gender priorities right side up.

DHEA To The Rescue

Even when pure testosterone becomes available in a form that makes it possible to synchronize it with the rhythm of the hormone cascade, dosage will be critical. End organ sex hormones are wild and woolly. It doesn't take much of an excess to spin you out of control. There is a better, safer way further up the cascade. DHEA is an intermediate steroid produced by the adrenals. It acts mainly as a substrate for more active hormones. One hormone your body can make readily from DHEA is testosterone.

Female bodies can make oodles of testosterone from DHEA in heart, skin, body fat, and brain, and in postmenopausal ovaries. As you will see in the DHEA chapter, female adrenal production of DHEA drops dramatically at perimenopause, one reason why her testosterone level also drops. Supplemental DHEA restores it nicely.

You don't have to use much DHEA. In one recent study, 150 mg per day of oral, micronized DHEA increased testosterone levels four-fold: 300 mg increased levels seven-fold in postmenopausal women.[17]

You don't need that much. Dr. Samuel Yen and colleagues at the University of California, San Diego, have shown repeatedly that 25 - 50 mg of DHEA per day, is sufficient to double testosterone levels in postmenopausal women.[18] That's enough.

Best of all, these small doses of DHEA do not appear to provoke any negative feedback to the brain, because they don't affect secretion of luteinizing hormone, follicle stimulating hormone or prolactin from the pituitary gland.[19] Nor do they cause other detrimental side-effects. Especially when used in conjunction with melatonin, this recent evidence recommends DHEA, as a safe and easy way to restore female testosterone.

24

Hormonal Nutrition

Scientists used to believe that human flesh required only a handful of essential nutrients, all of them large and obvious, **oxygen** and **hydrogen** from the air, **nitrogen, carbon** and **sulfur** from meats, **starches** and **sugars** from grains, vegetables and fruits. The prevailing dogma of medicine for 200 years was that fresh air and a good mixed diet provided everything you need for health.

Hoary old lies are hard to kill. When British naval physician, Dr. James Lind first proposed that tiny amounts of a chemical in limes and oranges are essential to prevent the disease of scurvy, that then decimated ship's crews, he was laughed out of the Royal Society of Medicine. It took another 48 years before the evidence prevailed, and British sailors were issued limes as part of their daily diet. Scurvy disappeared and with its much healthier navy of "Limies", Brittania ruled the waves.

Now we know that chemical as **ascorbic acid (vitamin C).** It is classified as a "vitamin" because your body can't make it. Vitamin C is essential for the health of our mucous membranes and connective tissue, and has wide-ranging antioxidant functions throughout the body.[1]

When Japanese researcher Kanehiro Takaki published evidence in the medical journal **Lancet**, that the then common disease of beri-beri was caused by a nutritional deficiency, he was ridiculed.   Thirty-five years later biochemist Casimir Funk isolated the vitamin **thiamin (vitamin B₁)** and beri-beri became history.

In 1968, solemn pronouncements of the American Academy of Sciences dismissed the mineral **chromium** as unnecessary for human nutrition.[2] By 1980 the evidence prevailed, and chromium was given its rightful place as essential for insulin metabolism.[3]

Delayed by similar pomposity, it look 35 years before selenium was allowed into the American Recommended Dietary Allowances in 1989.[4] Other nutrients well accepted as essential by science, **pantothenic acid, molybdenum, boron, co-enzyme Q10, essential fatty acids**, and certain **flavonoids** still wait to make the official list.

Vitamin Concept Obsolete

Government thinking on nutrition is stuck in the obsolete past.   In the '50s **lipoic acid**, for example, was being considered as an addition to the B-vitamins. But because your body can make it, and does so every day, it did not qualify as a true vitamin and never made the list.

Exclusion of lipoic acid, and of many other substances from the list of essential nutrients, brings me to an important advance in nutrition science that you must understand in your quest for hormonal health. "Vitamin" is a crude and now obsolete concept, used to describe "essential nutrients" which the human body cannot make, but must obtain from food. It assumes that if your body can make even a tiny amount of a chemical, then it doesn't need to get it from outside.

The pursuit of "vitamins" was reasonable 50 years ago, when biochemistry was not sufficiently advanced to determine biological needs. Now we know there are many substances the body can make, but cannot make enough for optimal health.

Your body makes the amino acids arginine, and carnitine, for example, but in increasing numbers of disorders it doesn't make enough, and patients require supplementation. Clinging to the old concepts, some medicine men now call these amino acids "conditionally essential," as illogical a piece of gobbledegook as you could find.

The new science of nutrition recognizes that there are many substances that do not fall under the old "vitamin" rubric, which are nevertheless essential, and must be obtained from your nutrition, because your body cannot make them in sufficient quantities to maintain itself.

As you read this, thousands of scientists including myself, are fighting to persuade old men who, by their refusal to die, have risen to positions of power that guard the nutrition dogma of the past. Their influence continues to damage the health of millions of Americans.

Out of interest, I recently qualified as a dietitian at New York State University, and passed the state licensing requirements. The official policy is still that our normal diet contains sufficient of all the vitamins, minerals, and other nutrients, and that a good mixed diet is all you need for health. Hogwash and flapdoodle!

Nutrient Needs

My book **The New Nutrition** analyzes the government studies and medical research showing that Americans are deficient even in many of the officially accepted nutrients, that our food is degraded, and that our food, water and air are heavily polluted. If you believe otherwise then read that book as a primer to this one.[5]

If you already know the truth, then I feel confident in stating boldly that hormonal health requires regular supplies of more than 60 chemicals that your body cannot make in sufficient amounts, or cannot make at all. You have to get them from your nutrition.

You cannot miss out even one of them, because all nutrients work in synergy with each other in the trillions, yes trillions of complex chemical reactions that go on in your body every second of your life. **It is the multiple interactions of**

nutrients, not their single actions, which form the basis of all biological functions.

I cover the science behind the synergy of nutrients, and the ratios and amounts of each required in previous books.[5-7] Suffice here to give you a couple of basic examples. Vitamin E deficiency also depletes your body of zinc, despite ample zinc in your diet. When E is low, zinc pinch-hits for some of its functions, thereby raising your zinc requirement. Without sufficient zinc to control it, body levels of copper then increase to cause all sorts of toxic mischief.[8]

Another example is vitamin B6, which a recent government study showed was deficient in 80% of a representative sample of 38,000 Americans.[9] Vitamin B6 deficiency impairs vitamin B2 metabolism which, in turn, impairs folic acid metabolism. Folic acid dysfunction then impairs vitamin C metabolism, which then reduces body absorption of iron, which allows excess copper absorption, which impairs zinc metabolism, and on and on and on.[10]

Taking account of all such findings known to science, the Colgan Institute has evolved a multi-vitamin/mineral antioxidant supplement, that forms the micronutrient base of all our nutrition programs. This formula stems from our 22 years of research into human performance and longevity. It deserves study. Whenever you buy a multi-nutrient supplement, make sure it contains every substance named in the table below, and in similar amounts. The intellectual, emotional, and physical benefits that flow from its regular use are extraordinary.

Multi-Vitamin/Mineral Basic Formula

Fat Soluble Vitamins

A (retinol)	7,500 IU	E (d-alpha tocopherol)	400 IU
Beta-carotene	12,500 IU	K (phylloquinone)	75 mcg
D3 (cholecalciferol)	400 IU		

Water Soluble Vitamins

B1 (thiamin)	50 mg	Biotin	500 mcg
B2 (riboflavin)	45 mg	Folic Acid	400 mcg
B3 (niacinamide)	80 mg	C (calcium ascorbate)	250 mg
B3 (niacin)	50 mg	C (magnesium ascorbate)	100 mg
B5 (pantothenic acid)	150 mg	C (ascorbic acid)	250 mg
B6 (pyridoxine)	50 mg	C (ascorbyl palmitate)	150 mg
B12 (cobalamin)	100 mcg		

Essential Fatty Acids

Linoleic acid	150 mg	Alpha-linolenic acid	250 mg
Gamma-linolenic acid	25 mg		

Accessory Nutrients

Phosphatidylserine	180 mg	Lipoic acid	100 mg
Phosphatidyl choline	200 mg	Pinus epicatechins	10 mg
Inositol	200 mg	Grape procyanadins	65 mg
Coenzyme Q10	30 mg	Grape seed flavonoids	100 mg
Para-amino-benzoic		Proanthocyanadins	120 mg
acid (PABA)	35 mg	Phenols and indoles	900 mg
Lutein	6 mg	Ginkgo biloba extract	80 mg
Lycopene	15 mg	Citrus flavonoids	250 mg

Minerals

Calcium (carbonate)	800 mg	Copper (gluconate)	500 mcg
Magnesium (aspartate)	600 mg	Chromium (picolinate)	200 mcg
Potassium (aspartate)	100 mg	Selenium	
Zinc (picolinate)	15 mg	(selenomethionine)	200 mcg
Iron (picolinate)	10 mg	Iodine (potassium iodide)	100 mcg
Manganese (gluconate)	6 mg	Molybdenum (trioxide)	60 mcg
Boron (aspartate)	3 mg		

Antioxidants: The Bottom Line

Antioxidants are big news. Twenty years of multiple controlled studies, show that they protect the body from diseases as diverse as atherosclerosis, diabetes and cancer.[5] The evidence is so strong that renowned but conservative scientists, such as Professor Meir Stampfer and Walter Willett of Harvard University are publicly recommending them in national media. In March 1994, eminent government scientist Dr. Jeffrey Blumburg, of the USDA Human Nutrition Research Center, said it right, "We have the confidence that these things really do work."[5]

Despite this huge advance in prevention of disease, most people I have asked, and all journalists and radio and television hosts who have interviewed me, have little idea what antioxidants are or how they work. Here is the bottom line. Oxidation is the most powerful process of decay on Earth. The rusting of steel, the rotting of meat, the hardening of arteries all take place by oxidation. One year after the new Statue of Liberty was completed, and protected by every means known to science, the American Institute of Architects reported to Congress that it was already being eaten away by oxidation.

Your body is similarly damaged. The brain is made mostly of fat and feeds on sugar and oxygen. This explosive combination creates a mass of oxidation that can cause widespread damage. With usual aging, this damage silently accumulates, until the basic structures of the brain no longer function properly.

The brain damage shows itself initially as forgetfulness and emotional blunting, then as progressive degeneration of memory, intelligence, positive emotions, hormones, and even simple motor movement. The trembling of Parkinson's and the senility of Alzheimer's, are graphic end points of cumulative brain damage that begins to take hold of Mr. and Mrs. Average in their thirties. To avoid this brain decline you need to know about bodily oxidation and how to prevent it.

To dip into a smidgen of physics, oxidation is caused by free radicals, that is, unstable atoms or molecules, usually of oxygen, which have an unpaired electron whizzing around the nucleus, instead of the usual stable pairs of electrons. This unstable nuclear configuration creates an electomagnetic force, which sucks an electron out of the nearest stable molecule. This molecule then becomes a new free radical. The chain reaction of damage multiplies until every material we know, steel, glass, granite, and human flesh disintegrate to dust.

Unless it is stopped. Your body makes powerful antioxidants, such as **glutathione, catalase, and superoxide dismutase**, that neutralize free radicals. Without them you would die in a heartbeat. But we know from the last 30 years of research, spearheaded by Dr. Denman Harman at the University of Nebraska, that the body cannot make enough antioxidants to completely protect itself.

So we add nutrient antioxidants to help. I cover these in detail in previous books.[5-7] Suffice here to provide a table below of the nutrient antioxidants and the amounts we use at the Colgan Institute. The lower end of the ranges provides reasonable figures for an antioxidant program to support hormonal health.

Antioxidants used in medical studies and studies with athletes.

Nutrient	Daily Amount
N-acetyl cysteine *	50 - 350 mg
L-glutathione	100 - 200 mg
Vitamin A (palmitate)	5000 - 10,000 IU
Beta-carotene **	10,000 - 25,000 IU
Vitamin C as:	
ascorbic acid	2000 - 10,000 mg
calcium ascorbate	500 - 1000 mg
magnesium ascorbate	500 - 1000 mg
ascorbyl palmitate	250 - 500 mg
Vitamin E as:	
tocopherol complex	200 - 800 IU
d-alpha tocopheryl succinate	400 - 1200 IU
Zinc (picolinate) §	10 - 60 mg
Selenium ‡ as:	
selenomethionine	200 - 400 mcg
sodium selenite	100 - 200 mcg
Co-Enzyme Q10	30 - 60 mg

* N-acetyl cysteine should be used only with at least three times its amount of vitamin C, so as to avoid the possibility of it precipitating in the kidneys as cysteine, and possibly causing kidney stones in sensitive individuals.

** Beta-carotene is a safe source of vitamin A at the levels given. Vitamin A may become toxic beyond 25,000 IU per day.

§ Zinc acts as an antioxidant co-factor.

‡ Selenium can become very toxic over 800 micrograms per day, especially in the inorganic form of sodium selenite.

Source: Colgan Institute, San Diego, CA

L-Arginine for Hormones

In addition to the basic formula, the **Hormonal Health Program** focuses on certain nutrients that act specifically to maintain the hormone cascade. Scientists used to believe that the amino acid **L-arginine** was essential only for growth in children. Now we know better. Studies during the last five years show that L-arginine is essential to provide the nitrogen for supplies of the biochemical **nitric oxide, (NO)**. NO is now known to have multiple functions throughout the body, from control of blood pressure to penile erection, and vaginal sexual arousal.[11] Arginine is so effective at stimulating these hormonally controlled responses, that some researchers advocate L-arginine as an aphrodisiac.

In women, nitric oxide levels depend on complex interactions between L-arginine and estrogen.[12] In both sexes L-arginine acts to increase growth hormone. Supplementary L-arginine in multi-gram amounts, taken last thing at night increases growth hormone release.[13] It also prevents inhibitory effects on the hormone cascade of the stress hormone **cortisol**.[14]

The main problem with using multi-gram amounts of L-arginine is that it raises body ammonia levels and also promotes growth of herpes viruses. So if you have any form of herpes, beware.[7]

At the Colgan Institute, for anyone who has even mild lip herpes, we advise **ornithine alpha-ketoglutarate (OKG)**, which is an ammonia-free source of the amino acid **ornithine**. Ornithine does not promote herpes and is readily converted to arginine in your body. OKG also stimulates the hormone cascade by other mechanisms, because it raises body glutamine levels.[6] With many programs we use a combination of 5 grams L-arginine and 5 grams OKG, taken at night 2 hours distant from protein food.

Get your Potassium

Potassium is an essential nutrient for both your brain and your hormone cascade, because it is the main **cation** (positively charged electrolyte) in your cells. It interacts with sodium and chloride to conduct all your nerve impulses. With insufficient potassium available, everything slows down. No surprise then that animals deprived of adequate potassium, show a 50% drop in growth hormone and IGF-1.[15]

Potassium deficiency also reduces testosterone levels to near zero in animals, though the mechanism is unknown. Potassium supplementation promptly restores their potency.[16]

Humans get insufficient potassium and too much sodium, especially on the typical highly processed diet. Fresh, unprocessed food contains much more potassium than sodium. Even seafood from a sodium-rich environment has more potassium.

Fresh tuna, for example, contains 100 parts potassium to 20 parts sodium. During processing this natural ratio is reversed. Canned tuna is 330 parts sodium to 100 parts potassium.[6] Natural butter has little sodium. Processed, salted butter has a whopping 3,600 parts sodium to 100 parts potassium.

This unnatural ratio of electrolytes causes all sorts of mischief, from raised blood pressure, to kidney problems, to reduced hormone levels. Don't take a lot of potassium as supplements. If you want hormonal health, ditch the salt and salty processed foods, in favor of fresh, potassium-rich foods uncontaminated by the machinations of man.

Zinc Your Hormones

Zinc forms part of many enzymes in your body, involved in thousands of different functions from cell growth to testosterone production. Your body pool of zinc is small and easily compromised.

Studies of American adults show an average zinc intake of only 8.6 mg.[17] Zinc deficiency is so widespread that some researchers suggest it is one cause of the astronomical rise in male impotence and female frigidity in America.[18] Recent studies showed, that even one month of zinc deficiency reduced male testosterone levels by 20%. Zinc supplementation promptly restored the hormone.[19] Make sure you get yours.

Chromium Your Hormones

Throughout this book the hormone insulin has come up repeatedly in discussions of growth hormone, estrogen, testosterone and the brain controls of the whole hormone cascade. In the '70s, Dr. Walter Mertz of the US Dept. of Agriculture, Human Nutrition Research Center, showed conclusively, that the mineral chromium is essential for optimal insulin metabolism.

Chromium used to be abundant in our food, but it is easily destroyed by processing. From sugar cane to white sugar for example, over 90% of the chromium disappears.[20] Because of modern food processing and storage, chromium is now scarcer than hens' teeth. Despite an official recommended intake of 50 - 200 micrograms per day, average chromium intake in America has fallen to about 25 micrograms.[20] That makes chromium one of the most deficient essential minerals in the US food supply.

Considerable evidence indicates that the upper limit of the recommended chromium allowance is too low to maintain hormonal health.[5-7] At the Colgan Institute we advise an average of 400 micrograms of **chromium picolinate** per day with all **Hormonal Health Programs**. Numerous studies show that this form of chromium is safe and effective in maintaining insulin metabolism[6], and thereby can help maintain the balance of your whole hormone cascade.

A further hormonal benefit of chromium picolinate deserves mention. Anti-diabetic drugs which improve insulin metabolism also raise DHEA levels.[21] I would not advise their use, however, because of toxic side-effects. There are no studies yet to prove it, but I will stick my neck out and predict that chromium picolinate should show a similar benefit for DHEA. And it will do the trick without any side-effects at all.

Boron Is Essential

Decades of animal studies show, that deficiency of the mineral boron stunts the bone growth of animals, but no one knew how. Then, in 1990, Dr. Forrest Nielson at the USDA

Human Nutrition Research Center gave postmenopausal women a diet low in boron (250 micrograms per day) for four months. Their already low estradiol and testosterone levels dropped through the floor. Then he added 3 mg of boron per day for 7 weeks. Both estradiol and testosterone jumped back up again.[22]

Some seamy sports supplement companies have used these findings to deceive athletes, claiming that boron will raise their testosterone levels. No way. Studies of boron supplementation in athletes show no effects whatsoever.[23] Nevertheless, the evidence from menopausal women suggests that the mineral may be essential for hormonal health.

Further studies by Nielson and colleagues show that boron supplements produce some of the beneficial changes of estrogen replacement therapy, and also enhance effects of estrogen, with no toxicity and no side-effects.[24] At the Colgan Institute we advise 1 - 3 mg of boron per day in all female **Hormonal Health Programs** and in many male programs, especially where there is evidence of estrogen decline.

Lipoic Acid For Nerves

Your brain is particularly vulnerable to free radical damage because of its high oxygen consumption. To maintain your hormone cascade you should do everything possible to protect it. One of our criteria for selection of substances to include in the **Hormonal Health Program**, was strong antioxidant activity. Melatonin, selegiline and acetyl-L-carnitine all display potent action against brain free radicals.

To up the ante even more, we also use 100 - 200 mg per day of **alpha-lipoic acid**.

We became interested in lipoic acid, (also called thiotic acid), in the '70s, when European physicians began using it to treat the nerve degeneration of diabetes.[25] It has particular actions in preventing what is called **glycation** damage.

Glycation is a process whereby the interaction of sugar, proteins, and oxygen form waste products, much like the clinker in a boiler. This clinker builds up in all of us and is one way that we age, because it progressively interferes with brain and organ function. Diabetics, because of their abnormal sugar metabolism, are especially subject to glycation damage.[26] I am indebted to Dr. Lester Packer, world expert on antioxidants, for showing how lipoic acid has unique antioxidant actions against glycation.[26]

Smart Fats

Each of your brain cells is enclosed in a fatty membrane that controls the continual flow of chemicals in and out of the cell. All this traffic takes place by specific chemical transport systems. Except for these systems, the cell membrane is leakproof. It remains leakproof only if you provide a continuing supply of repair and maintenance materials. These consist of vitamins, minerals and mainly essential fatty acids, which your body cannot make, but must obtain from your nutrition. Only two fats are essential, **linoleic acid**, the start of the omega-6 series, and **alpha-linolenic acid**, the start of the omega-3 series. From these your body can make all the rest.

Because of human meddling, undamaged essential fatty acids have become sadly deficient in the food supply throughout Western Society. For the sake of your brain, it's important to understand how this deficiency came about. A little peek at the biochemistry, will enable you to see both the magnificence of Nature's design, and the clumsy human meddling that has rendered most fats unfit to eat.

All fats and oils consist of fatty acids, arranged in sausage-like chains of carbon atoms with hydrogen atoms attached to them. Different fats have different length chains. In Nature, the hydrogen atoms are all on the same side of the carbons, in what is called a **cis** configuration. Because of their electromagnetic charge, the hydrogens repel each other, causing the chain to adopt a series of U-shaped bends. These humps and hollows are the precise keys that fit the chemical locks in your brain to make healthy, leakproof brain cell membranes.

The **cis** configuration of most fats and oils is destroyed by modern processing methods including boiling, hydrogenation, bleaching and deodorizing. These man-made "improvements" to natural oils, add hydrogen atoms and also rotate some of the existing hydrogen atoms, so they now lie on opposite sides of the carbon chain. This is called a **trans** configuration. It is very unhealthy, because the carbon chain of fats in a trans configuration straightens out in places where the opposing hydrogen charges cancel each other. Bingo! They lose the humps and hollows that form the precise keys of Nature's design.

Your brain still tries to use these damaged fats, but because they don't fit properly, the cell membranes leak and function poorly or not at all.

I am giving you this information in detail, because most of the public are still unaware of the unhealthy nature of almost all cooking oils, margarines and oil products. Goods with high levels of trans fats are already being banned by the European Community, but American oil industry lobbies have so far squashed attempts to change American oils. Use them at your peril, because recent studies have implicated trans fats in numerous diseases, including cardiovascular disease and cancer.[5]

At the Colgan Institute we use virgin olive oil which is unprocessed, and organic flax oil. You can get all the essential fatty acids you need from about a teaspoon of flax oil a day. Barleans and Arrowhead Mills are two reliable brands. If you want your brain to continue to support your hormones -- use them.

One final point. With usual aging, your ability to produce an enzyme called **delta-6-desaturase** declines. This enzyme converts linoleic acid into the next step in the omega-6 chain, **gamma-linolenic acid**. For nutritional insurance we use 100 - 200 mg of gamma-linolenic acid per day with many of our programs. The best sources are borage or blackcurrant oils, or the more expensive evening primrose oil.

Phosphatidylserine For Smarts

In your brain cell membranes, some essential fatty acids are arranged in a configuration called **phosphatidylserine**, a mixture of phosphorus and fat, mostly fat. Phosphatidylserine oversees a multitude of tasks. It stimulates release of brain neurotransmitters, it activates transport of nutrients, and it regulates glucose availability.

Much of the brain activity involved in memory and learning is dependent on continuous adequate levels of phosphatidylserine.[27,28]

Phosphatidylserine levels decline with usual aging. After age 25, you are on the downward slope. Some researchers suggest that this decline underlies the increasing difficulty of learning new material as you age.[29,30]

In May 1981, I and my labmates ran around Rockefeller University shouting "Eureka." We had just received new Italian research, showing that a supplemental form of phosphatidylserine improved memory and learning in aged rats. A pristine memory, and the ability to learn rapidly, are the pearls of a researcher's existence. Even back then, 25 years ago, we knew that all the nutrition, all the supplements, all the exercise, come to naught unless you can protect the functions of your brain cell membranes. Surrounded by doddery old professors, who demonstrated every day that they had lost the ability to think, we were very aware of our own mortality.

At that time, the phosphatidylserine was being laboriously extracted from cow brains and cost a bundle. Nevertheless, we were determined to get enough for research, and for ourselves. Right on the brink of bankrupting our research grants, the bad news broke. Despite spectacular results in rejuvenation of brain function, some of the rats were dying of **spongiform encephalopathy**. Some batches of the phosphatidylserine were carrying a stowaway, a slow virus that causes "mad cow disease." That was the end of that.

In 1990 the whole picture changed. The Lipogen company succeeded in making vegetable phosphatidylserine from

Savoy cabbages and soy lecithin.   By 1992, they were manufacturing a commercial product that was both inexpensive and completely safe. We were back in business to save our membranes.

To date there are only animal studies with the vegetable compound, but bovine phosphatidylserine has improved brain function in numerous studies of human senility.[31-34] In a representative test of the new vegetable compound, baby mice were given phosphatidylserine from birth to sixty days old, and compared with a control group. At one month, the supplemented mice showed higher intelligence than control mice. At two months, the supplemented mice learned faster and more accurately than adult mice.[35]   After a quarter century of research, I think the evidence is now sufficient to warrant addition of 100 - 200 mg of vegetable phosphatidylserine "brain saver" to our daily supplements.

Good Food

None of the aforementioned supplements will work well unless you first fix your food. I cover healthy diets in detail in previous books.[5-7] Use my book, **The New Nutrition** especially as a guide to the diet for hormonal health.[5] To put it in a nutshell here, avoid fats, avoid sugar, avoid processed carbohydrates, avoid junk-food. Use coffee, cola, chocolate, and other caffeine containing foods very moderately, all to total no more than the equivalent of three cups of coffee a day.   Eat a high-fiber, low-acid diet, emphasizing low glycemic index foods. See the table of combined low-glycemic, low-acid foods below.

Low Acid/Low Glycemic Index Foods

Especially Eat These	Eat These Moderately		Avoid These Foods	
Low-acid Low-glycemic	Moderately-acid Moderately-glycemic (steamed/roasted/dried)		High-acid High-glycemic (fried/sautéed)	
Drinks	**Drinks**		**Drinks**	
Water	Black tea	Green tea	Beer	Red wines
Mineral water	Herbal teas	White wine	Orange juice	Cocoa
Grapefruit juice				
	Meats		**Meats**	
Vegetables	Turkey	Ocean fish	Beef	Chicken
Broccoli			Lobster	Mussels
Diakon	**Vegetables**		Pork	Veal
Endive	Azuki beans	Fava beans	All fatty meats	
Garlic	Kidney beans	Navy beans		
Kale	Pinto beans	String beans	**Vegetables**	
Kohlrabi	Wax beans	Carrots	Soybeans	Peas
Lentils	Cauliflower	Chard	Chickpeas	Potatoes
Lotus root	Eggplant	Lettuce		
Mustard greens	Pumpkin	Squash	**Fruits**	
Onions	Tomatoes		Oranges	
Peppers				
All sea vegetables	**Fruits**		**Grains**	
Sweet potatoes	Apples	Apricots	Rye	Maize
Yams	Blueberries	Cherries	Corn	Puffed rice
	Figs	Grapes	White bread	White rice
	Guava	Oranges	Corn chips	Potato chips
	Pears	Plums	Rice cakes	Puffed wheat
	Strawberries		Instant rice	French bread

Low Acid/Low Glycemic Index Foods (Cont'd)

Especially Eat These	Eat These Moderately		Avoid These Foods
Low-acid Low-glycemic	Moderately-acid Moderately-glycemic (steamed/roasted/dried)		High-acid High-glycemic (fried/sautéed)
Fruits	**Grains**		**Dairy**
Black berries	Amaranth	Barley	All cheese Butter
Cantaloupe	Buckwheat	Kasha	Casein (milk protein)
Grapefruit	Pasta	Quinoa	
Honeydew	Brown rice	Wild rice	**Oils/Fats**
Limes	Spelt	Oatmeal	Cottonseed Palm
Loganberries	Whole wheat spaghetti		Palm kernel
Nectarines			
Raspberries	**Dairy**		**Sweets**
Tangerines	Cow's milk	Goat's milk	Table sugar Glucose
Watermelon	Chicken eggs	Duck eggs	Hard candy Raw sugar
	Goat cheese	Yogurt	Chocolate Carob
Other			Jams Jellies
Soy sauce	**Oils/Fats**		Ice Cream Aspartame
Cinnamon	Flax oil	Canola oil	All candy bars
Sea salt	Olive oil		
			Nuts
	Sweets		Brazils Hazels
	Honey (unrefined)		Pecans Walnuts
	Maple syrup (unrefined)		
			Other
	Other		Antibiotics
	Tofu	Umeboshi	
	Balsamic vinegar		

Source: Colgan Institute, San Diego, CA.

Plan your food so that proteins form 25-30% of the diet, carbohydrates form 45-55%, and fats form 15-20%. Get almost all your fats as **cis**-form essential fatty acids by using virgin olive oil and organic flax oil with salads, and other foods, and as a supplement.

Eat Less

Most of us eat far too much because of the social and emotional needs fulfilled by food. **The Hormonal Health Program** is an excellent regulator of appetite. It will help you to eat only in response to genuine hunger. Eating less is a proven way to maintain brain dopamine metabolism.[36]

Nevertheless, don't go on any calorie-restrictive diets. As I have shown elsewhere, repeated use of such diets makes you fatter.[5] If you adopt a **Hormonal Health Program**, you should find yourself gradually becoming slimmer, and then remaining that way for life.

Organic Foods

I cover in previous books the contamination and destruction of many of our foods with pesticides, herbicides, hormones, antibiotics and detrimental processing.[5-7] To avoid their low levels of nutrients and the bodily pollution they carry, we try to eat only organic, unprocessed, drug-free food. Over the last two decades, thousands of research groups including the Colgan Institute, have kept up relentless pressure to restore natural foods. We have had heartening success. Now, almost anyone in America can obtain organic produce, drug-free meats, and clean water, even from their local supermarket.

If you want hormonal health you will take full advantage of this blessing. Leave the poisonous and processed products on the store shelves. The most powerful vote in America is that of the pocketbook. Exercise it well and the polluted, nutritionless pap will gradually disappear, and with it a lot of the man-made disease and degeneration that now plagues our lives.

Pure Water

Don't make the error of doing everything else and then drinking and using water from the faucet. I document elsewhere the deplorable state of American drinking water.[2,3] The water supply systems are so out of date and decrepit there is a disease disaster from contamination somewhere in America every month. Suffice here to note just the latest catastrophe recorded this week, 10 April 1996, in the **Journal of the American Medical Association.** In August 1995, the Idaho Department of Health reported an outbreak of *Shigella sonnei* in their well water. This organism is the main cause of dysentery in the United States.[37]

Drink only distilled water preferably from a home distiller, so you can trust it. For the last decade we have used in-line systems from the Pure Water company in Lincoln, Nebraska. They form part of our hidden plumbing, and operate automatically, much like your water heater. They produce water so pure I can use it in laboratory procedures. Your deserves the same degree of purity. Remember, even Rush Limbaugh is 70% water.

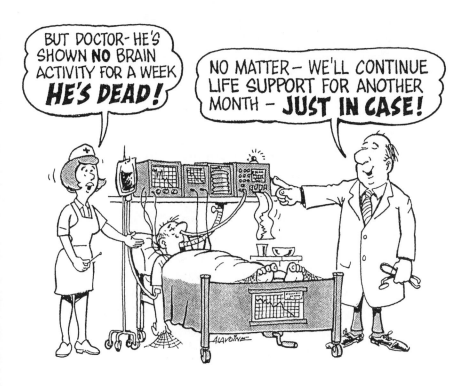

Hormonal Exercise

In 1982 Dr. Walter Bortz of the Palo Alto Medical Clinic in California, reviewed over 100 studies, showing that the sedentary lifestyle of Americans causes widespread bodily damage.[1] Since then, a mass of research supports his conclusions that couch potatoism sets up chain reactions of decay.[2,3]

First it reduces **vital capacity**, your body's ability to take up and use oxygen. Then it reduces **cardiac output**, the amount of blood pumped by your heart. You get a double-whammy of deprivation, less oxygen, and less blood to carry essential nutrients to your brain and organs. Blood pressure rises in a vain attempt to feed the brain. Sex hormones decline, muscles shrink, bones thin, minds fog. The TV couch destroys health faster than you know.

An excellent study by Dr. Ken Cooper and colleagues, at his Aerobics Center in Dallas, shows the end result. They followed 13,344 men and women for 15 years. Death from all causes, even including accidents, was strongly linked with inactivity.[4] ***Disuse is deadly.*** Let's look at a few examples of its effects on your hormones.

Exercise Your Bones

Your bones are constantly remodeled throughout life under the dual influences of hormones, and the stresses placed on them by weight-bearing activity. Bone is like a living honeycomb. Each day it sheds millions of worn out bits of the structure. In order to make replacements to maintain structural integrity, your muscles have to contract sufficiently hard to stress each junction point of the bone honeycomb. The stress triggers an electrochemical "spark" which sets in motion complex chemistry of estrogen (and progesterone) to model new bone. This chemistry creates a synergy of the minerals calcium, magnesium, zinc, copper, manganese, fluoride, silica, and boron, plus vitamin D.[5] Now you know why the popular calcium supplements are a complete failure in maintaining bone.[3]

Aerobic exercise will not maintain your bones either. Without sufficient pressure, there's no electrochemical spark. No spark, no bone. Scientists didn't really appreciate the necessity for weight-bearing exercise until men went into space. Despite daily aerobic exercise, they came back with accelerated loss of bone, because there was no gravity pressure to maintain it.[6]

Representative studies show that aerobic exercise done on Earth also fails miserably to maintain bone.[7] In contrast, weight exercise can even reverse bone loss.[8] In a typical study of postmenopausal women, a year of aerobic exercise yielded almost a 4% *loss* of bone. When weight training was added over the next two years, the loss was reversed and the women showed a net *gain* of bone.[9] Without weight-bearing exercise, your body cannot use its hormones properly to protect your bones.

Muscle Is Your Engine

Much of the current epidemic of osteoporosis in Western Society, occurs because of the decline in weight-bearing work. With labor-saving everything, our habitual activity no longer maintains sufficient muscle mass to effectively stimulate bone growth. And if we have insufficient muscle to maintain bone, you can bet your boots we have insufficient to perform the muscular activities that maintain the hormone cascade.

Between ages 20 and 80, the average man in Western society loses a quarter of his total muscle mass.[10] His weight, however, goes up not down, because he puts on more than enough fat to match the muscle loss. Women show the same pattern. Between ages 20 and 40 the average American woman loses 8 lbs of muscle and gains 23 lbs of fat.

Even most of the folk who exercise regularly do not maintain their muscle, because the predominant forms of exercise are aerobic, walking, jogging, cycling, swimming, and aerobics classes. Properly done, aerobic exercise has proven benefits for heart and lungs, and forms a vital part of our **Hormonal Health Program.** But it fails utterly to maintain muscle.

President Clinton is a good example. Surrounded by the most expensive medical advisors money can buy, he jogs 3 miles a day 5 days a week. Though not yet 50 years of age, his sockfuls of pudding legs have become a national joke.

His exercise regimen, for which earlier monarchs would have had their advisors beheaded, doesn't even keep the fat off, or protect his heart. Figures quoted by national media from his annual physical in 1995, show that the President has gained 6 lbs in a year, and his elevated cholesterol of 203 mg/dl, hasn't budged. Doesn't bode well for his hormones.[11]

Latest reports from Michael McCurry the White House press secretary, are that Mr. Clinton is starting a weight training program. It's a move in the right direction, but if the program advised is anything like his faulty jogging program, there's little chance of an extended presidential lifespan.

A good weight training program can do wonders for both muscle and fitness. In a typical study, Dr. Neil McCartney and colleagues at McMaster University in Ontario, compared 2½ hours of aerobic exercise per week for 10 weeks, against 2½ hours split between aerobics and weight training. The aerobics group showed only a 2% increase in cardiovascular capacity and an 11% increase in endurance. The aerobics plus weights group showed a 15% increase in cardiovascular capacity and a massive 109% increase in endurance.

More important, the aerobics group showed zero increases in strength. The aerobics plus weights group showed strength increases in different muscles ranging from 21% to 43%.[12] The judicious combination of aerobic exercise plus weight-bearing exercise is the key, both for strength and aerobic fitness.

Exercise For Brains

The dopamine receptors in the striatal cortex decline with usual aging with consequent decline of memory, cognition and the whole hormone cascade.[13] Aerobic fitness can slow that decline. Numerous animal studies show that rats rewarded for doing exercise programs, show increases in dopamine receptor numbers and activity.[14,15]

New studies now show similar effects in humans. Dr. Hoau-Yan Wang and colleagues at the Medical College of Pennsylvania in Philadelphia, have just published the latest study, comparing groups of men aged 20 - 36 and 61 - 78. They measured an enzyme called **protein kinase C**, a sensitive indicator of brain function that declines rapidly with brain aging. They found that the older men who exercised regularly maintained enzyme activity similar to that of young men. Older sedentary men showed low enzyme activity and other signs of brain degeneration.[16] For the sake of your dopamine system, exercise lifelong.

Muscle Your Growth Hormone

As we move down the hormone cascade, a ton of recent research shows that growth hormone is also linked to exercise and fitness. In a representative study, Drs. Eric Poehlman and Kenneth Copeland at the University of Vermont, College of Medicine, measured the amount of physical activity and the VO_2 max of healthy, young and old men. At all ages, those who exercised regularly as part of their leisure time activity, had higher levels of VO_2 max, and higher levels of insulin-like growth factor 1 (IGF-1), the test usually used to measure growth hormone activity.

Bodyfat provided another important indication that fitness maintains growth hormone. As I showed you in a previous chapter, maintaining growth hormone is one way to keep the fat off. In the Poehlman study, fit subjects of all ages had much lower levels of bodyfat.[17]

The type of exercise is also important. Numerous studies show that progressive weight training is the most reliable exercise to increase growth hormone output in both young and old men.[18]

Recently, Dr. Bill Kraemer and colleagues at Penn State University have shown that the form of weight exercise is also important.[19] They gave one group of men and women a program of sets of 5 repetitions with heavy weights and long rest periods between sets. This is the best form of weight training for gains in absolute strength or power. They gave another group sets of 10 repetitions with less weight and short rest periods between sets. This is the best form of weight training for strength plus endurance.

Growth hormone increases were much greater with the 10-repetition program in both males and females, indicating the importance of an endurance or fitness component in weight training for hormonal health.

Exercise Your Testosterone

Exercise also affects testosterone levels. Although numerous studies show a decline in testosterone with usual aging, more detailed analyses that eliminate the sick and sedentary from the samples, show that fit and active old men maintain testosterone levels in the youthful range. Men who are unfit show lower testosterone levels at all ages.[20]

As with growth hormone, the type of exercise is also important. Though it's a popular fad for ordinary folk to run marathons for fitness, it's not a good idea for hormonal health. Running (or cycling) long distances, and other forms of exhaustive aerobic exercise, are reliably linked to *reduced* testosterone levels in males, even in elite athletes.[21-23] In women athletes, exhaustive endurance training *lowers* estrogen levels.[24] It's fine to run, cycle, and swim for fitness, but don't fall in the trap that more is better.

Weight training seems to have only beneficial effects on testosterone. In the Kraemer study above, male subjects showed large increases in testosterone levels.[19] Not any old weight training will do, however. At the Colgan Institute we compared minor muscle stress using light dumbbells in an aerobics class, against heavy muscle stress of the back and legs using weight machines. Testosterone rose significantly only with the heavy exercise. Bill Kraemer agrees. "To get a rise in testosterone, you have to activate major muscles like the quadriceps, hamstrings, and pectorals."[25]

Dr. Morris Notelovitz, at the Women's Medical and Diagnostic Center in Gainsville, Florida is an expert in exercise programs for menopausal women. His exercise prescription matches ours and Bill Kraemer's. He starts with weight training the large muscles. Like Kraemer, he finds that sets of 8 - 10 repetitions with a one minute rest between them are best.[26]

Ecstatic Exercise

Another link between exercise and hormonal health is the effect of exercise on emotions. We have seen already how incidence of depression rises sharply in women at perimenopause and thereafter. In men depression and emotional blunting are more variable, but nevertheless increase in incidence with usual aging.

As the hormone cascade declines, regular exercise provides a non-toxic, treatment that is far more successful than any man-made medications. In a typical study, 6,000 average Americans were followed from 1965 to 1983. Those engaging in regular, moderate or high-level physical activity had a much lower risk of depression than sedentary subjects.[27]

Even a short exercise program can make a difference. In one study of students, a single bout of exercise reduced their levels of both anger and anxiety.[28]

Over a period of weeks, results can be dramatic. In a typical study of depressed women, subjects chose to be enrolled in an aerobics class. They were compared with similarly depressed subjects in a psychology class. After 10 weeks, only the aerobics subjects showed a significant reduction in depression.[29]

Everyone has heard of the elusive **endorphins** produced by exercise, opiate-like chemicals in the striatal cortex, that produce feelings of elation and euphoria by their interactions with brain neurotransmitters and hormones.[30] It's likely that exercise stimulates positive emotions by lightly tapping into the hormonal roots of ecstacy.

Starting To Exercise

First, see your physician for approval. Then, *START EASY*. Most folk who begin to exercise after a long lay-off, do far too much. If you haven't exercised for a year or more, initially your body will stand only 20-30 minutes of light exercise, three times a week. More than that leads to pains, strains, and injuries and the give-up reaction.

I see it repeated every year. Each Spring, hordes of lumpy men and women enter the gym with a roar, flashing multi-colored "underwear", New Year determination, and jaw-clenched smiles. After a few weeks of thrashing themselves, they vanish with a whimper, ne'er to be seen again until Spring next year.

Before you begin any exercise program fix this information in your memory. The proteins in your muscles take a minimum of six months to turn over once. Much of your bone is renewed only once a year. To have a permanent effect, you have to exercise regularly for at least that long. Anything less is mostly a waste of time.

So set up a program you know you can stick with. Thirty minutes, three mornings a week is enough to start, and far better than a 3-hour exhausting grind on Saturdays.

Your body will tell you when to increase. If you sleep better and rise refreshed, if your waking pulse gradually falls, if you dodge colds and flus while all about you sniffle and snort, if you find new spring in your step and laughter in your heart, only then should you up the ante.

Exercise Programs

I cover the evidence for different types and methods of exercise programs in previous books.[2,3,31] Here I will give you only the details. The **Hormonal Health Exercise Program** achieves three results that will help you maintain the hormone cascade and all its benefits. First, you will increase muscle and strength. Second, you will increase endurance and fitness. Third, you will increase flexibility, essential to avoid the pains and strains.

Once you have your physician's clearance to exercise in this way, write your own program card, so you can record progress. Begin with a column for aerobics. Each exercise session should start with light aerobics for two reasons. First, it allows the heart and arteries to get into action without an undue strain. Second, it loosens the muscles and increases the blood flow, to offset the risk of injury from a large muscular effort.

At the Colgan Institute we use walking or jogging on a treadmill for 20 - 40 minutes, with speed and duration depending on your starting level of fitness. Beginners walk 20 - 30 minutes at 3.5 miles per hour.

At the finish of aerobics you should be nice and sweaty. The rule is: ***Never touch a weight until you break a sweat.*** That way we stay injury-free year round.

The weight work should be divided into three sessions minimum to five sessions maximum per week, depending on your starting level of fitness. Except in advanced programs, don't exercise more than two days in a row. For a 4-session weekly program, we advise two days on, one day off, two days on, two days off.

Rest Days Are Essential

You gain muscle and strength only during sleep or rest, never during exercise. It takes a lot of rest for maximum gains. After a weight session, muscle takes about two days to break down and dispose of wastes, then another two to three days to grow the replacement tissues. After that it maintains new strength for about another three days. So you should wait 5 - 8 days before repeating any particular exercise. Popular programs that I see in gyms, where exercises are repeated two or three times in a week, are next to useless.

A 3-day per week program for hormonal health consists of:

Day 1	Shoulders and Arms
Day 2	---
Day 3	Chest and Back
Day 4	---
Day 5	Legs and Abdominals
Days 6 and 7	---

A 4-day per week program consists of:

Day 1	Shoulders
Day 2	Arms and Abdominals
Day 3	---
Day 4	Chest and Back
Day 5	Legs
Days 6 and 7	---

A 5-day per week program consist of:

Day 1	Shoulders
Day 2	Arms and Abdominals
Day 3	Chest
Day 4	---
Day 5	Back and Abdominals
Day 6	Legs
Day 7	---

Sets and Reps

You do not need to spend hours in the gym. A good program consists of only 9 - 12 sets per session. Each weight session should take no more than 30 - 40 minutes. Beyond that is self-defeating and can *reduce* your hormone levels.

Both standard and advanced exercises that you can do at home with little or no equipment, or in the gym with fancy machines are described in detail in my book **The Power Program**.[31] But simple exercises are all you need to begin.

If you have little or no experience with weights, then I strongly advise that you go to a good gym and have a couple of sessions with a certified trainer. If you are in Southern California or can get there, the Frogs Gyms have the best training available anywhere. If not, call us at (619) 632-7722 for a home video program. Trainers will teach you the correct form of the movements. Unless you do each movement correctly, you not only court injury, but may make little or no progress. Some basic but good exercises are:

Shoulders	**Arms**
Lateral Dumbbell Raise	Barbell Curl
Overhead Dumbbell Press	Alternate Dumbbell Curls
Dumbbell Front Raise	Tricep Chair Dips
Bent-Over Dumbbell Raise	Kickbacks
Chest	**Back**
Push Ups	Pull Ups (Chins)
Barbell Bench Press	Bent-Over Barbell Rows
Incline Dumbbell Press	One-Arm Dumbbell Rows
Legs	**Abdominals**
Squats	Hanging Knee Kicks
Leg Extensions	Lying Crunches
Leg Curls	
Lunges	

Do three sets of each exercise. (four sets for advanced programs). All sets are to exhaustion.

First set, use a weight with which you can do 12-15 repetitions. At 12 repetitions you should be starting to fail. If you have a workout partner, *a very good idea*, they will have to help you with the last 2-3 reps.

Second set is your strength set. Set the weight so you can do 6-8 repetitions, to exhaustion. You should be starting to fail on rep 6.

Third set, for advanced programs only is, the power set The weight used permits only 4-6 repetitions. You should be failing on rep 4.

Third and last set for most programs is also the last set for advanced programs. It aims to increase the capillary growth in your muscles, to increase their blood supply, and their capacity for endurance. Set the weight for 20 - 25 reps. You should be starting to fail at about rep 15.

When you have been exercising with weights for at least six months, you can incorporate a variation that will increase your gains. **To do this before you have exercised regularly for six months will only lead to injury.** For every rep of every exercise, accelerate the concentric contraction and decelerate the eccentric contraction. That is, quicken the movement when your muscles are shortening under load, for example, when curling a barbell up to your chest. Then slow the movement right down when the muscle is lengthening under load, for example, when you are lowering the weight in the barbell curl.

Flat Abdominals

The only exceptions to sets and reps are the abdominals. Many exercise programs cause the abdominals to grow and protrude. You want your abdominals to get smaller and tighter. That way they will support your organs in the correct position lifelong. One help in achieving this goal is to consciously pull in your abdominals at the start of every set of every exercise.

You also need a good abdominals program. Don't do traditional sit-ups. Don't do Roman chairs. Don't do leg raises. All are failures for the abs. Instead, do knee kicks to your chest while hanging on a bar. Do as many as you can non-stop. Keep your back rounded throughout. Don't swing. If you find yourself swinging you are using other muscles than the abs, and the exercise becomes ineffective.

As soon as you drop from the bar, lie on your back with knees up and legs half bent, arms across chest. Crunch your abs by raising your head and shoulders off the floor, while pushing the small of your back into the floor. Do as many as you can non-stop. This basic abs program will serve you well for at least a year. Then you are ready for the more advanced work given in my book **The Power Program**.[31]

Flexibility

Immediately after each weight session do some light stretching. Excellent stretches are given by the basic movements of Hatha Yoga. It's worthwhile attending a yoga session at your local gym to learn the movements correctly.

Some basic rules for flexibility.

1. Whenever you stretch, you should be warm and sweaty.

2. Never bounce. Move smoothly.

3. Never force or strain.

4. Relax your muscles thoughout the movements.

5. Breathe easily from the belly thoughout the movements.

6. Patience. Flexibility takes years to accomplish. Every time you force it, you inhibit progress.

Remember, never undertake an exercise program without your physician's approval of that program. Exercising, especially with weights, is not an innocuous activity. It is a powerful way to change your body which can easily lead to injury. Nevertheless, most of the 35,000 people who have taken programs from the Colgan Institute over the last two decades have found nothing but benefit. Even if you have not exercised for thirty years, with the first rep of the first set on the first day, your body will start to rejuvenate.

26

The Way To Go

When I first proposed the **Hormonal Health Program** to medical and scientific colleagues in 1985, none questioned the scholarship but many were aghast. Typical comments were: "It seems so unnatural, why not just eat right and let Nature take its course?" "Why fight it? You are going to age and die anyway." "Seems an awful lot of trouble to gain a few years."

All of the men and women who made such comments are now on **Hormonal Health Programs**, and enthusiastic and grateful about the health benefits they have experienced. Nevertheless, such criticisms are common and deserve an answer.

Is It Unnatural?

We wear artificial clothes of nylon and polyester that never existed in Nature. We drive and fly in vehicles of plastic and unnatural metals. We communicate in cyberspace. We drink from polystyrene cups, chemical sodas that never saw the light of ancient suns. We eat food so processed that it will resist the natural rot of real food, to lie unchanged for years on supermarket shelves. We see through plastic lenses in our eyes, fill the holes in our teeth with unnatural compounds, and put steel struts in our hips. We live today in an unnatural world.

If anything, the **Hormonal Health Program** is closer to Nature than most of the rest of our lives. It attempts to keep the body healthy by using Nature's rhythms, Nature's nutrients and compounds. To extend your health and your lifespan by *preventing* disease and degeneration, is far less artificial than to use man's motley mix of toxic medicines, surgery, and prostheses, to try to keep your ailing body alive *after* it has been ravaged by disease.

You Are Going To Die Anyway

So many times I have had sick folk referred to me who have little time left to live, who will pay and do anything to extend that time by even a few months. It is easy for the hale and hearty to dismiss the **Hormonal Health Program** as irrelevant to their lives. But, once mortality has tapped them on the shoulder, they often become fervent converts.

I always keep in mind one day in 1982, when well known writer Barry Stevens came to the clinic for celebrities, which I ran before I got more sense, in a large medical complex of plastic surgeons and cosmetic dentists on Sunset Boulevard in Hollywood. A very fine old lady, she had had a stroke and was partially paralyzed, sick and depressed. She could not speak intelligibly but her nurse/companion told me, "All she wants is enough time to finish her last book."

Within three months we had her walking, talking, and full of life. She finished the book **Burst Out Laughing,** did a six-month world tour, and added another three years to her very long life of love and laughter with her children and grand-children.

If you begin early enough, a good **Hormonal Health Program** could extend vital healthy life by as much as 30 years. If that's not the greatest prize on Earth, then your slant upon this mortal coil is very different from mine.

Seems A Lot of Trouble

At first glance the **Hormonal Health Program** does look complex. But once you get it going, it doesn't intrude on life at all.

It's no more trouble to take the packet of vitamins, minerals and other compounds every morning and evening, than it is to clean your teeth. It's no more trouble to buy good food, than it is to buy bad food. Once you get a little fit, it's no more trouble to exercise, than it is to sit TV crazydreaming.

Basic Programs

I cannot stress enough that these programs are only a guide for your physician.   You should not undertake any **Hormonal Health Program** without the advice and approval of your physician.   These are powerful manipulations of your body, and only your own physician can provide the essential testing and interpretation to adapt them to your unique bodily needs.

Program Components

1. The **vitamin/mineral/antioxidant formula** given in the nutrition chapter, taken half with breakfast and half with dinner.

2. **Melatonin** at 1.0-3.0 mg per day taken last thing at night.

3. **Acety-L-carnitine** at 500-2000 mg per day, taken first thing each morning.

4. **Selegiline hydrochloride** at 1.0-3.0 mg five mornings per week, taken first thing.

5. **DHEA** at 25-50 mg per day five mornings per week, taken first thing.

6. For women who have reached perimenopause: the **Tri-Est** formula of estrogen given in the chapter on estrogen therapy, plus 0.1 to 0.3 mg pure **testosterone** via patch or cream.

Only for men who have documented testicular degeneration: the **Androderm** patch discussed in the chapter on male testosterone.

7. For women who have reached perimenopause the **progesterone cream** discussed in the chapter on progesterone.

8. For both men and women, the combined **aerobic, weight training, and flexibility program** discussed in the chapter on exercise.

I am writing this in Miracles Coffee Bar, in Cardiff-By-The-Sea north of San Diego. With the best coffee in Southern California, it has become a haunt of elite athletes, students and beach boys. Surrounded by the health and beauty of youth, I am saddened that the commercialization of medicine has produced an industry that relies on the continuing growth of disease to maintain its profits. This "sickness industry" has inhibited the development of programs such as mine, which would enable the mass of citizens to extend their youth and beauty, and avoid many of the ravages of aging.

But I am happy to tell you that most of the concepts in this book are not mine, but come from the work of thousands of scientists worldwide. I have been able to sketch for you only a fraction of the evidence supporting our conclusions. But I am not a lone voice, simply a herald of the coming revolution in medicine.

And when it comes to the inevitable public fight between the purveyors of pharmaceutical poisons and the champions of natural health, we are well prepared. It's my hope that the battle will be bloodless, and that those commercial forces who control the medical industry will yield gracefully. Then they can employ the very scientists who oppose them, to design systems of hormonal health which will overflow their coffers with the gold of Midas.

More important, these new systems of medicine, which will act in concert with Nature instead of against her, will prolong healthy human life beyond our wildest dreams.

Come, play with me for extended vitality and health in the new millennium.

References

Chapter 1: Chemical Castration

1. Impotence: NIH Concensus Conference. **J Amer Med Assoc**, 1993;270:83-90.

2. Kolberg R. Human embryo cloning reported. **Science**, 1993;262: 652-653.

3. Kirby RS, et al. **Impotence.** Oxford: Butterworth-Heinemann, 1991.

4. **New York Times**, 7 July 1995.

5. Wagner G, Singer Kaplan H. **The New Injection Treatment for Impotence.** New York: Brunner Mazel, 1993.

Chapter 2: Female Repression

1. Kinsey AC, et al. **Sexual Behavior in the Human Female.** Philadelphia: WB Saunders, 1953.

2. Reiss I. **Journey into Sexuality.** Englewood Cliffs, NJ: Prentice-Hall, 1986.

3. Singer Kaplan H. Sex, intimacy and the aging process. **J Amer Acad Psychoan**,1990;18:185-205.

4. Denney NW, Quadagno D. **Human Sexuality.** St. Louis: Mosby College Publishing, 1988.

5. Swerdloff RS, Wang C. Androgens and aging in men. **Exper Gerontol**, 1993;28:435-446.

6. **Physicians Desk Reference, 49th Edition.** Montvale NJ: Medical Economics, 1995.

7. Bancroft J, et al. Oral contraceptives androgens and the sexuality of young women. **Arch Sexual Behav**, 1991;20:121-35.

8. Herzberg BN. Oral contraceptives depression and libido. **Brit Med J**, 1971;3:495-500.

Chapter 3: All In Your Head

1. Anthony CP, Thibodeau GA. **Textbook of Anatomy & Physiology.** St. Louis: CV Mosby, 1983.

2. Rosen RC, Ashton AK. Prosexual drugs: Empirical status of the "new aphrodisiacs." **Arch Sexual Behav,** 1993;22:521-543.

3. Everitt BJ. Sexual motivation: A neural and behavioral analysis of the mechanisms underlying appetite and copulatory responses of male rats. **Neurosci Biobehav Res,** 1990;14:217-232.

4. Everitt BJ, Bancroft J. Of rats and men: The comparative approach to male sexuality. **Ann Rev Sex Res,** 1991;2:77-118.

Chapter 4: Sex & Emotions

1. Sem-Jacobsen CA. **Depth Electrographic Stimulation of the Brain and Human Behavior.** Springfield: Thomas, 1968.

2. Colgan M. **Optimum Sports Nutrition.** New York: Advanced Research Press, 1993.

3. Robinson BW, Mishkin M. Penile erection evoked from forebrain structures in Macaca Mulatta. **Arch Neurol,** 1968;19:184-198.

4. Yen S, Jaffee R. **Reproductive Endocrinology.** Philadelphia:WB Saunders, 1978.

5. Persky H, et al. The relation of plasma androgen levels to sexual behaviors and attitudes of women. **Psychosom Med,** 1982;44:305-319.

6. Mooradian AD, et al. Biological action of androgens. **Endocrin Rev,** 1987;8:1-28.

7. Kidd GS, et al. The hypothalamo-pituitary-adrenal-testicular axis in thryrotoxicosis. **J Clin Endocrin Metab,** 1979;48:798-801.

8. Milward DJ, et al. Role of thyroid, insulin and corticosteroid hormones in the physiological regulation of proteolysis in muscle. **Prog Clin Biol Res,** 1985;180:531-542.

9. Milward DJ, et al. **J Endocrinol,** 1988;118:417-422.

10. Hellman L, Bradlow HL. Recent advances in human steroid metabolism. **Advances in Clin Chem**, 1970;13:1-25.

11. Bouloux PM, Wass JAH. Endocrinology. In Kirby RS, et al. **Impotence,** Oxford:Butterworth/Heineman, 1991, 44-54.

12. Prescott RW, et al. Hyperprolactimnia in men: Response to bromocriptine therapy. **Lancet,** 1982;1:245-249.

13. Seagraves RT. Hormones and libido. In Lieblum RS, Rosen RC (eds), **Sexual Desire Disorders.** New York: Guilford, 1988.

14. Schiavi RC, et al. Healthy aging and male sexual function. **AM J Psychiat,** 1990;147:776-771.

15. Larson L. **Acta Physiol Scand,** 1978;36 (S):457.

16. Kinsey AC, et al. **Sexual Behavior in the Human Male.** Philadelphia:WB Saunders, 1948.

17. Kinsey AC, et al. **Sexual Behavior in the Human Female.** Philadelphia:WB Saunders, 1953.

18. Martin CD. Martial and sexual factors in relation to age, disease, and longevity. In Wirdt RD, (eds). **Life History Research in Psychopathology, Vol. 4.** Minneapolis: University of Minnesota Press, 1975.

19. Singer Kaplan H. Sex intimacy and the aging process. **J Am Acad Psychoan,** 1990;18:185-205.

Chapter 5: Orgasm

1. Michael RT, et al. **Sex in America: A Definitive Survey,** New York:Little Brown, 1994.

2. Singer Kaplan, H. Sex intimacy and the aging process. **J Am Acad Psychoan,** 1990;18:185-205.

3. Wagner G, Singer Kaplan H. **The New Injection Treatment for Impotence.** New York: Brunner Mazel, 1993.

4. Bancroft J, et. al. Oral contraceptives androgens and the sexuality of young women. **Arch Sexual Behav,** 1991;20:121-35.

5. Rome E. **Our Bodies, Ourselves,** 1ˢᵗ ed., New York: Simon & Schuster, 1973.

6. Lief HI. Sexual survey #36: Current thinking on the orgasm experience. **Med Aspects Hum Sex**, 1980;14:55-62.

7. Colgan M. **The New Nutrition: Medicine for the Millennium,** Vancouver: Apple Publishing, 1994.

8. Colgan M. Just a wee squeeze please. **Muscular Development,** 1994, January.

Chapter 6: Hormones For Smarts

1. Parlee MB, Menstrual rhythms in sensory processes: A review of fluctuations in vision, olfaction, audition, taste and touch. **Psychol Bull**, 1983;93:530-548.

2. Coyle JT, et al. Alzheimer's disease: a disorder of cortical cholinergic innervation. **Science**, 1983;219,1184-1190.

3. Bartus RT, et al. The cholinergic hypothesis of geriatric memory dysfunction. **Science**, 1982;217:408-414.

4. Luine V. Estradiol increases choline acetyltransferase activity in specific basal forebrain nuclei and projection areas of female rats. **Exper Neurol**, 1985;89:484-490.

5. Luine V, et al. Immunochemical demonstration of increased choline acetyltransferase concentrations in rat preoptic area after estradiol administration. **Brain Res**, 1980;191:273-277.

6. Sohrabi F, et al. Estrogen differentially regulates estrogen and nerve growth factor receptor in RNAs in adult sensory neurons. **J Neurosci**, 1994;14:459-411.

7. Honjo H, et al. Estrogen as a growth factor to central nervous cells. Estrogen treatment promotes development of acetylcholine-stearase-positive basal forebrain neurons transplanted in the anterior eye chamber. **J Steroid Biochem Mol Biol**, 1992;41:633-635.

8. Sherwin B, Kampen D. Estrogen use and verbal memory in healthy postmenopausal women. **Obstet Gynecol**, 1994;83:979-983.

9. Robinson D, et al. Estrogen replacement therapy and memory in older women. **J Amer Geriat Soc**, 1994;42:919-922.

10. Sherwin BB, Phillips S. Estrogen and cognitive functioning in surgically menopausal women. **Ann NY Acad Sci**, 1990;592:474-475.

11. Halbreich V, et al. **Proceedings of the International College of Neuropsychopharmacology Meeting**. Washington DC, July 1994.

12. Sherwin BB. Estrogenic effects on memory in women. **Ann NY Acad Sci**, 1994;743:213-231.

13. Schellenberg GD, et al. Genetic linkage evidence for a familial Alzheimer's disease locus on chromosome 14. **Science**, 1992;258:668-671.

14. Levy-Lahad E, et al. Candidate gene for the chromosome 1 familial Alzheimer's disease locus. **Science**, 1995;269:973-977.

15. Marott Sinex F, et al (eds). **Alzheimer's Disease, Down's Syndrome, and Aging**, New York: New York Academy of Sciences, 1982.

16. Rocca WA, et al. Epidemiology of clinically diagnosed Alzheimer's disease. **Ann Neurol**, 1986;19:415-424.

17. Colgan M. **The New Nutrition: Medicine for the Millennium.** Vancouver: Apple Publishing, 1994.

18. Christiansen K, Knussman R. Sex hormones and cognitive functioning in men. **Neuropsychobiology**, 1987;18:27-36.

19. Janowsky JS, et al. Testosterone administration enhances spatial cognition in older men. **Soc Neurosci Abstracts**, 1991;16:340:12

20. **Endocrine Society**, 1995 Annual Meeting, Washington DC, June 1995.

21. Forssell LG, et al. Early stages of late onset Alzheimer's disease. IV. Biochemical measurements suggesting metabolic derangement. **Acta Neurol Scand**, 1989;79:Suppl:67-86.

22. Amaducci LA, et al. Risk factors for clinically diagnosed Alzheimer's disease: a case control study of an Italian population. **Neurology**, 1986;36:992-931.

23. Paganini-Hill A, Henderson VW. Estrogen deficiency and risk of Alzheimer's disease in women, **Amer J Epidemiol**, 1994;140:256-261.

24. Pettigrew JW, et al. Clinical and neurochemical effect of acetyl-l-carnitine in Alzheimer's disease, **Neurobiol Aging**, 1995;16:1-4.

25. Salvioli NM. L-acetyl carnitine in treatment of mental decline in the elderly, **Drugs Exptl Clin Res**, 1994;20:169-176.

26. Spagnoli A, et al. Long-term acetyl-l-carnitine treatment in Alzheimer's disease, **Neurology**, 1991;41:1726-1732.

27. Hellegoarch A, et al. **Gen Pharmacol**, 1985;16:129.

28. Clostre F, DeFeudis FV. **Cardiovascular Effects of** *Ginkgo biloba* **Extract (EGB761),** New York: Elzevier, 1995.

29. Cross AJ, et al. Reduced dopamine beta-hydroxylase activity in Alzheimer's disease. **Brit Med J**, 1981;282:93-94.

Chapter 7: Hormones and Emotions

1. Robins LN, Regier DA, (Eds.). **Psychiatric Disorders in America: The Epidemiologic Catchment Area Study,** New York: Free Press, 1991.

2. Orn HS, et al. Design and field methods of the Edmonton Survey of Psychiatric Disorders. **Acta Psychiatr Scand**, 1988;338:17-23.

3. Lepine JP, et al. **Psychiatr Psychobiol**, 1989;4:267.

4. Wittchen HU, et al. Lifetime and 6-month prevalence of mental disorders in the Munich follow-up study. **Eur Arch Psych Clin Neurosci**, 1992;241:247-258.

5. Faravelli C, et al. Epidemiology of Mood Disorders: a common survey in Florence. **J Affective Disord**, 1990;20:135-141.

6. Wells JE, et al. Christchurch Psychiatric Epidemiology Study, Part 1: methodology and lifetime prevalance for specific psychiatric disorders. **Aust NZJ Psychiatry**, 1989;23:315-326.

7. Wolk SI, Weissman MM. **Review of Psychiatry**, American Psychiatric Press, Washington DC 1995, vol. 14, chapter 9.

8. O'Hara MW, et al. Prospective study of postpartum blues, biologic and psychosocial factors.**Arch Gen Psychiatry**, 1991;48:801-806.

9. American Psychiatric Association Work Group on Major Depressive Disorder, **Am J Psychiatry**, 1993;150:Suppl 1-26.

10. Kendell RE, et al. Epidemiology of puerperal psychosis. **Br J Psychiatry**, 1987;150:662-673.

11. Martin CJ, et al. Psycho-social stress and puerperal depression. **J Affective Disord**, 1989;16:283-293.

12. Dr. Charles Grossman Immunoendocrinologist at Cincinnati's Veterans Administration Medical Center. Personal Communication, 25 September 1995.

13. Schreiner-Engel P, Schiavi RC. Lifetime psychopathology in individuals with low sexual desire. **J Nerv Ment Dis**, 1986;174:646-651.

14. Hawton K, et al. Long term outcome of sex therapy. **Behav Res Ther**, 1986;24:665-675.

15. De Amicis LA, et al. Clinical follow-up of couples treated for sexual dysfunction. **Arch Sex Behav**, 1985;14:467-489.

16. **Endocrine Society**, 1995 Annual Meeting, Washington DC, June 1995.

17. Brenner WJ, et al. **J Clin Endocrin Metab**, June 1994.

18. Catalan J, et al. Couples referred to a sexual dysfunction clinic. Psychological and physical morbidity. **Brit J Psychiat**, 1990;156:61-67.

19. Warner P, Bancroft J. A regional clinical service for psychosexual problems: A three-year study. **Sex and Marital Ther**, 1987;2:115-126.

20. Osborn M, et al. Sexual dysfunction among middle-aged women in the community. **Brit Med J**, 1988;296:959-962.

21. Garde K, Lunde I. Female sexual behavior: A study in a random sample of 40-year-old women. **Maturitas**, 1980;2:225-240.

22. Frank E, et al. Frequency of sexual dysfunction in "normal" couples. **New Engl J Med**, 1978;299:111-113.

23. Longcope C, et al. Steroid and gonadotropin levels in women during the peri-menopausal years, **Maturitas**, 1986;8:189-196.

24. Rannevik G, et al. A prospective long-term study in women from pre-menopause to post-menopause: Changing profiles of gonadotropins, oestrogens and androgens. **Maturitas**, 1986;8:297-307.

25. Longcope C. Hormone dynamics at the menopause. In Flint M, et al (eds). **Multidisciplinary Perspectives on Menopause**, New York: New York Academy of Sciences, 1990, 21-30.

26. **The Metpath Reference Manual**, Teterboro NJ: Metpath, 1995.

27. **Physicians Desk Reference: 49ᵗʰ Edition**. Montvale, NJ: Medical Economic, 1995, p. 2727.

28. Karlsberg J, et al. A quality of life perspective on who benefits from estradiol replacement therapy. **Acta Obstet Gynecol Scand**, 1995;74:367-372.

29. Sherwin BB. Affective changes with estrogen and androgen replacement therapy in surgically menopausal women. **J Affective Dis**, 1988;14:177-187.

30. Kirby RS, et al (eds). **Impotence**. Oxford: Butterworth-Heinemann, 1991.

31. Martin CE. Sexual activity in the aging male in Money J, Musaph H (eds). **Handbook of Sexology**, Amsterdam: Elsevier, 1977.

Chapter 8: Drugs Hit Hormones

1. Kirby RS, et al (eds). **Impotence,** Oxford: Butterworth-Heinemann, 1991.

2. Bouloux PM, Wass JAH. Endocrinology, in Kirby RS, et al (eds). **Impotence**, Oxford: Butterworth-Heinemann, 1991, 44-54.

3. Impotence: NIH Consensus Conference, **J Amer Med Assoc**, 1993;270:83-90.

4. Singer Kaplan, H. Sex intimacy and the aging process. **J Am Acad Psychoan**, 1;18:185-205.

5. Segal S, et al. Male hyperprolactinemic effects on infertility. **Fertility and Sterility**, 1979;32:556-559.

6. Prescott RW, et al. Hyperprolactinemia in men-response to bromocriptine therapy. **Lancet**, 1982;1:245-249.

7. Papadopoulous C. Cardiovascular drugs and sexuality. **Arch. Int. Med.**, 1980;140:1341.

8. Balon R, et al. Sexual dysfunction during antidepressant treatment. **J Clin Psychiat**, 1993;54:209-212.

9. **Patterson WM. Fluoxetine-induced sexual dysfunction.** J Clin Psychiat, **1993;54:71.**

10. **Medical Tribune**, 18 May 1995, 13.

11. Steiner M, et al. Fluoxetine in the treatment of premenstrual dysphoria. **New Engl J Med,** 1995;332:1529-1534.

12. Chopra IJ, Tulchinsky D. Status of estrogen-androgen balance in hyperthyroid men with Graves' disease. **Journal of Clinical Endocrinology,** 1974;38:297-301.

13. Kidd GS, et al. The hypothalamo-pitiutary-adrenal-testicular axis in thryrotoxicosis. **J Clin Endocrin Metab,** 1979;48:798-801.

14. Hellman, L, Bradlow, HL. Recent advances in human steroid metabolism. **Advances in Clin Chem,** 1970;13:1-25.

15. Schurmeyer T, et al. The relationship of lipoprotein(a) (Lp(a)) to risk factors of coronary heart disease: Initial results of the prospective epidemiological study on company employees in Westfalia. **Journal of Clinical Chemistry and Clinical Biochemistry,** 1984;22:591-596.

16. Matsumoto AM, Brenner WJ. Parallel dose-dependent suppression of LH, FSH, and sperm production by testosterone in normal men. **Abstract No. 570, Proceedings of the 70th Annual Meeting of the Endocrine Society,** 1988; The Endocrine Society, Bethesda, Maryland.

17. World Health Organization Task Force on Methods for the Regulation of Male Fertility, Contraceptive efficacy of testosterone-induced azoospermia in normal men. **Lancet,** 1990;336:955-959.

18. Wing TY, et al. Restoration effects of exogenous luteinizing hormone on the testicular steroidogenesis and Leydig cell ultrastructure. **Endocrinology,** 1985;117:1779-1787.

19. Martikainen H, et al. Testicular responsiveness to human chorionic gonadotropin during transient hypogonadotrophic hypogonadism induced by androgenic/anabolic steroids in power athletes. **Journal of Steroid Biochemistry,** 1986;25:109-112.

Chapter 9: That Pesky Pill

1. Seaman B. **The Doctors' Case Against The Pill,** PH Wyden, 1969.

2. Tomatis L (ed). Cancer, Causes, Occurrence and Control. World Health Organization International Agency for Research on Cancer. Patl. No 100, Lyon: WHO, 1990.

3. Former JG, Rhodes JE, (eds). **Accomplishments in Cancer Research,** Philadelphia: Lippincott, 1990.

4. Backstrom T, et al. Ovarian steroid hormones: effects on mood, behavior and brain excitability. **Acta Obstet Gynacol Scand,** 1985;Suppl;130:19-24.

5. Moline ML. Pharmacologic strategies for managing premenstrual syndrome. **Clin Pharm,** 1993;12:181-196.

6. Kaness FJ, et al. Mood and behavioral changes with progestational agents. **Brit J Psychiat,** 1967;113:265-268.

7. Meyerson B. Relationship between the anaesthetic and gestagenic action and estrus behavior inducing activity of different progestins. **Endocrinol,** 1967;81:369-374.

8. Squartini E, et al (eds). **Breast Cancer: From Biology to Therapy,** New York: NY Academy of Sciences, 1993.

9. **Johns Hopkins Medical Letter,** September, 1995, 6.

10. Colditz GA, et al. The use of estrogens and progestins and the risk of breast cancer in postmenopausal women. **New Engl J Med,** 1995;332:1589-1593.

11. Chilvers C, et al. Oral contraceptives and breast cancer risk in young women. **Lancet,** 1989;8645:973-982.

12. Olsson H, et al. Early oral contraceptive use as a prognostic factor in breast cancer. **Anticancer Res,** 1988;8:29-32.

13. Davis DL, Hoel D, (eds). **Trends in Cancer Mortality in Industrialized Countries,** New York: NY Academy of Sciences, 1990.

14. Colgan M. **Prevent Cancer Now,** San Diego: CI Publications, 1992.

15. Nilsson A, et al. Side-effects of an oral contraceptive with particular attention to mental symnptoms and sexual adaptation. **Acta Obstet Gynaecol Scand,** 1967;46:537-556.

16. Grounds D, et al. The contraceptive pill, side-effects and personality: Report of a controlled double blind trial. **Br J Psychiatr,** 1970;116:169-172.

17. Alexander GM, et al. Testosterone and sexual behavior in oral contraceptive users and non-users. **Horm Behav,** 1990;24:388-402.

18. Bancroft J, et al. Oral contraceptives, androgens, and the sexuality of young women: I. A comparison of sexual experiences, sexual attitudes, and gender role in oral contraceptive users and nonusers. **Arch Sex Behav**, 1991;20:105-120.

19. Herzberg BN, et al. Oral contraceptives, depression, and libido. **Br Med J**, 1971;3:495-500.

20. Graham CA, Sherwin BB. The relationship between mood and sexuality in women using an oral contraceptive as a treatment for premenstrual symptoms. **Psychoneuroendocrinology**, 1993;18:273-281.

21. Gibran K. **The Prophet**, New York:Alfred Knopf, 1973.

22. Michael RT, et al., **Sex in America: A Definitive Survey**, New York:Little Brown, 1994.

23. Harward M. Evaluation of sexual dysfunction in women. **Hosp Prac**, 1991, 15 October 53-57.

24. De Buono B, et. al. Sexual behavior of college women in 1975, 1986, and 1989. **New Engl J Med**, 1990;322:821-825.

25. Singer Kaplan H. Sex intimacy and the aging process. **J Am Acad Psychoan**, 1990;18:185-205.

Chapter 10: Prostate Problems

1. Hennenfont B. Prostatitis. **American Prostate Society Quarterly**, 1995;3:9.

2. Canadian Task Force on the Periodic Health Examination, 1991, Update 3: secondary prevention of prostate cancer, **Can Med Assoc J**, 1991;145:413-28.

3. Lawrence RS, US Preventive Services Task Force: **Screening For Prostate Cancer**, Washington DC: US Preventive Services, 1992, 1-23.

4. Johansson JE, et al, Natural history of localized prostate cancer, **Lancet**, 1989;15 April:799-803.

5. **Cancer Facts and Figures - 1994**, Atlanta, GA: American Cancer Society, 1994.

6. Krahn MD, et al, Screening for prostate cancer, **J Amer Med Assoc**, 1994;272:773-814.

7. Lu-Yao GL, et al. An assessment of radical prostatectomy: time trends, geographic location, and outcome, **J Amer Med Assoc**, 1993;269:2633-2636.

8. Albertson P. A 72-year old man with localized prostate cancer, **J Amer Med Assoc**, 1995;274:69-74.

9. Shipley WV, et al. Treatment related sequelae following external beam radiation for prostate cancer. **J Urol**, 1994;152:1799-1805.

10. Byar DP, et al. Hormone therapy for prostate cancer. **National Cancer Inst Monograph**, 1988;7:165-170.

11. Miller AB. Screening for cancer: state of the art and prospects for the future, **World J Surgery**, 1989;13:79-83.

12. Colgan M. **The New Nutrition: Medicine for the Millennium.** Vancouver: Apple Publishing, 1994.

13. Champault G, et al. A double-blind trial of an extract of the plant Serenoa repens in benign prostatic hypertrophy, **Br J Clin Pharm**, 1984;18:461-62.

Chapter 11: Hysterical Surgery

1. Easterday CL, et al. Hysterectomy in the United States. **Obstet Gynecol**, 1983;62:203-210.

2. National Center for Health Statistics, Hysterectomies in the United States. DHSS Publication No (PHS) 88-1753 Hyattsville MD: Public Health Service, 1988.

3. Pokras R, Hufnagel VG. Hysterectomies in the United States, 1965-1984. **DHSS Publication No (PHS) 87-1753**. Hyattsville MD: Public Health Service, 1987.

4. Coulter A, et al. Do British women undergo too many or too few hysterectomies? **Soc Sci Med**, 1988;9:987-994.

5. McPherson K, et al. Small area variations in common surgical procedures: An international comparison of New England, England, and Norway. **New Engl J Med**, 1982;307:1310-1314.

6. Bunker JP, Brown BW. The physician-patient as an informed consumer of surgical services. **New Engl J Med,** 1974;290:1051-1055.

7. Miller NF. Hysterectomy: Therapeutic necessity or surgical racket? **Am J Obstet Gynecol,** 1946;51:804-810.

8. Pratt JH. The unnecessary hysterectomy. **Southern Med J,** 1980;79:1360-1365.

9. Grant JM, et al. An audit of abdominal hysterectomy over a decade in a district hospital. **Brit J Obstet Gynecol,** 1984;91:73-77.

10. Amirikia H, Evans TN. Ten year review of hysterectomies, trends indications and risks. **Am J Obstet Gynecol,** 1979;134:431-437.

11. Wilcox LS, et al. Hysterectomy in the United States, 1988-1990. **Obstet Gynecol,** 1994;83:549-555.

12. Harris MB, Olive DL. Changing hysterectomy patterns after introduction of laparoscopically assisted vaginal hysterectomy. **Am J Obstet Gynecol,** 1994;171:340-344.

13. Wennberg JE, et al. Professional uncertainty and the problem of supplier induced demand. **Soc Sci Med,** 1982;16:811-824.

14. Amias AG. Sexual life after gynecological operations I. **Brit Med J,** 1975;2:608-609.

15. Lauersen N. **Listen to Your Body,** Los Angeles: Berkeley Books, 1983.

16. **Cancer Facts and Figures - 1994,** Atlanta, GA: American Cancer Society, 1994.

17. Garcia CR, Cutler WB. Preservation of the ovary: a re-evaluation. **Fertil Steril,** 1984;42:510-514.

18. Morell V. Zeroing in on how hormones affect the immune system. **Science,** 1995;269:773-775.

19. Charbomiet B, et al. Human cervical mucus contains large amounts of prostaglandins. **Fertil Steril,** 1982;38:109.

20. Cutler WB, et al. The psychoneuroendocrinology of the ovulatory cycle of women. **Psychoneuroendocrinology,** 1980;5:89-95.

21. Zussman L, et al. Sexual response after hysterectomy-oophorectomy. **Am J Obstet Gynecol,** 1981;140:725-729.

22. Kilkku P, et al. Supravaginal uterine amputation vs hysterectomy. Effects on libido and orgasm. **Acta Obstet Gynecol Scand,** 1983;62:147-152.

23. Sloan D. The emotional and psychosexual aspect of hysterectomy. **Am J Obstet Gynecol,** 1978;132:598-605.

24. Amias AG. Life after gynecological operations - II. **Brit Med J,** 1975;2:680-681.

25. Centerwall BS. Premenopausal hysterectomy and cardiovascular disease. **Am J Obstet Gynecol,** 1981;139:58-61.

26. Riedel HH, et al. Ovarian failure phenomena after hysterectomy. **J Reprod Med,** 1986;31:597-600.

27. Hreshchyshyn MM, et al. Effect of natural menopause, hysterectomy, and oophorectomy on lumbar spine and femoral neck bone densities. **Obstet Gynecol,** 1988;72:631-638.

28. Spector TD, et al. Increased rates of previous hysterectomy and gynecological operations in women with osteoarthritis. **Brit Med J,** 1988;297:899-900.

29. Lalinec-Michaud M, Engelesmann F. Depression and hysterectomy: A prospective study. **Psychosomatics,** 1984;25:550-558.

30. Kaltreider HB, et al. A field study of the stress response syndrome. Young women after hysterectomy. **J Amer Med Assoc,** 1979;242:1499-1503.

31. Denverstein L, et al. Sexual response following hysterectomy and oophorectomy. **J Nerv Ment Dis,** 1977;49:92-96.

32. Utian WH. Effect of hysterectomy, oophorectomy, and estrogen therapy on libido. **Int J Gynecol Obstet,** 1975;13:97-100.

33. Oldenhave A, et al. Hysterectomized women with ovarian conservation report more severe climacteric complaints than do normal climacteric women of similar age. **Am J Obstet Gynecol,** 1993;168:765-771.

34. Richards DH. A post-hysterectomy syndrome. **Lancet,** 1974;2:983-985.

35. Bickell NA, et al. Gynecologists sex, clinical beliefs and hysterectomy rates. **Am J Public Health,** 1994;84:1649-1652.

Chapter 12: Who Needs Hormones?

1. United Kingdom National Case Control Study Group. Oral contraceptive use and breast cancer risk in young women. **Lancet,** 1989;8643:973-978.

2. Hormone Therapy: Is it the right choice for you? **John Hopkins Medical Letter,** September 1995, 4-7.

3. **Time,** 26 June 1995, 45-52

4. Birnbaum D. Self-help for menopause. **Ann NY Acad Sci,** 1990;592:250-256.

5. **Woman's Health Advocate,** December 1995, 1-3.

6. Pearlstein TB. Hormones and depression. **Am J Obstet Gynecol,** 1995;173:646-653.

7. Hay AG, et al. Affective symptoms in women attending a menopause clinic. **Brit J Psychiat,** 1994;164:513-516.

8. Nachtigall L. **Estrogen: The Facts Can Change Your Life,** New York: Harper/Collins, 1994.

Chapter 13: Hormone Benefits

1. National Center for Health Statistics DHSS Publication Nos 88-1122 and 88-1114. Washington DC: OS Government Printing Office 1988.

2. U.S. Department of Health and Human Services, **Vital Statistics of the United States, Vol. II.** Hyattsville, MD: National Center for Health Statistics, 1988.

3. Gura T. Estrogen: Key player in heart disease among women. **Science,** 1995;269:771-773.

4. Colditz GA, et al. Menopause and the risk of coronary heart disease in women. **New Engl J Med,** 1987;316:1105-1110.

5. Flint M, et al. (eds). **Multidisciplinary Perspectives on Menopause,** New York: New York Academy of Sciences, 1990.

6. The Postmenopausal Estrogen/Progestin Intervention (PEPI) Trial, Affects of estrogen or estrogen/progestin regimens on heart disease

risk factors in postmenopausal women. **J Amer Med Assoc,** 1995;273:199-208.

7. **John Hopkins Medical Letter,** Hormone Therapy: Is it the right choice for you. September 1995, 4-6.

8. Bush TL. Non-contraceptive estrogen use and the risk of cardiovascular disease. In Korenman SG (ed), **Menopause,** New York: Plenum, 1992.

9. Doppelt S. **Harvard Medical School Newsletter,** November, 1981, 3-4.

10. Peek WA, et al. Research directions in osteoporosis. **Am J Med,** 1988;84:275-282.

11. Colgan M. **The New Nutrition: Medicine for the Millennium** Vancouver: Apple Publishing, 1994.

12. Albright F, et al. Postmenopausal osteoporosis. **Tr Assoc Am Phys,** 1940;55:298-305.

13. Aitken JM, et al. Osteoporosis after oophorectomy for non-malignant disease. **Brit Med J,** 1973;1:325-328.

14. Richelson LS, et al. Relative contributions of aging and estrogen deficiency to postmenopausal bone loss. **New Engl J Med,** 1984;311:1273-1275.

15. Lindsay R, Cosman F. Estrogen in prevention and treatment of osteoporosis. **Ann NY Acad Sci,** 1990;592:326-333.

16. Nachtigall L, Estrogen: The Facts Can Change Your Life, New York: Harper/Collins, 1994.

17. Barrett-Conner E, Laakso M. Ischemic heart disease risk in postmenopausal women. Effects of estrogen use on glucose and insulin levels. **Arteriosclerosis,** 1990;10:581-584.

18. Manson JE, et al. A prospective study of postmenopausal estrogen therapy and subsequent incidence of non-insulin dependent diabetes mellitus. **Ann Epidemiol,** 1992;2:665-673.

19. Lindheim SR, et al. A possible bimodal effect of estrogen on insulin sensitivity in postmenopausal women and the attenuating effect of added progestin. **Fertil Steril** 1993;60(4):664-667.

20. **Cancer Facts and Figures - 1994**, Atlanta, GA: American Cancer Society, 1994.

21. Screening for colorectal cancer. **J Amer Med Assoc,** 1996;275:830-831.

22. Newcomb PA, Storer BE. Postmenopausal hormone use and risk of large-bowel cancer. **J Natl Cancer Inst,** 1995;87:1067-1071.

23. Calle EE, et al. Estrogen replacement therapy and risk of fatal colon cancer in a prospective cohort of postmenopausal women. **J Natl Cancer Inst,** 1995;87:517-523.

24. Admirand WH, Small DM. The physico-chemical basis of cholesterol gallstones production in man. **J Clin Invest,** 1968;47:1043-1052.

25. Bruce WR, et al (eds.) **Gastrointestinal Cancer: Endogenous Factors,** New York: Cold Springs Harbor Lab 1981.

26. Bachmann GA. Sexual issues at menopause. **Ann NY Acad Sci,** 1990;592:87-94.

27. Detre T, et al. Management of the menopause. **Ann Intern Med,** 1978;88:373-378.

28. Berg G, et al. Climateric symptoms among women 60-62 in Linkoping Sweden. **Maturitas,** 1988;10:193.

29. **Time,** 26 June 1995.

30. Sarrel PM. Sex problems after menopause: A study of 50 married couples treated in a sex counselling program. **Maturitas,** 1982;4:231-237.

31. Maoz B, Durst N. The effects of estrogen therapy on the sex life of postmenopausal women. **Maturitas,** 1980;2:327-336.

32. Iwasaka T, et al. Hormonal status and mycoplasma colonization in the female genital tract. **Obstet Gynecol,** 1986;68:263-266.

33. Holland EF, et al. Changes in collagen composition and cross-links in bone and skin of osteoportic postmenopausal women treated with percutaneous estradiol implants. **Obstet Gynecol,** 1994;83:180-183.

34. Maheux R, et al. A randomized, double-blind, placebo-controlled study on the effect of conjugated estrogens and skin thickness. **Am J Obstet Gynecol,** 1994;170:642-649.

35. Pierard GE, et al. Effect of hormone replacement therapy for menopause on the mechanical properties of skin. **J Am Geriatr Soc**, 1995;43:662-665.

36. 1995 American Academy of Anti-Aging Medicine Conference, Las Vegas, Nevada, December 1995.

37. 10th Annual Meeting of the American College of Clinical Gerontology, San Antonio, Texas, October 1995.

38. Sarrel P, et al. Ovarian steroids and the capacity to function at home and in the workplace. **Ann NY Acad Sci**, 1990;592:156-161.

39. Coleman L, Antonucci T. Impact of work on women in middle life.**Dev Psychol**, 1983;19:290-295.

Chapter 14: Hormones Or Not

1. **Johns Hopkins Medical Letter**, Hormone Therapy: Is it the right choice for you. September 1995, 4-6.

2. **Physicians Desk Reference, 49th Edition.** Montvale NJ: Medical Economics, 1995.

3. Paroli E. Opioid peptides from food (the exorphins). **World Rev Nutr Dietet**, 1988;55:58-97.

4. Fukushima M, et al. Extraction and purification of a substance with luteinizing hormone releasing activity from the leaves of Avena sativa. **J Exper Med**, 1976;119:115-122.

5. Britton JR, Kastin AJ. Biologically active polypeptides in milk. **Am J Med Sci**, 1991;301:124-132.

6. Lamartiniere CA, et al. Neonatal genestein chemoprevents mammary cancer. **Proc Soc Exp Biol Med**, 1995;208:120-123.

7. Davis DL, Hoel D, (eds). **Trends in Cancer Mortality in Industrialized Countries**, New York: NY Academy of Sciences, 1990.

8. Flint M, et al. (eds). **Multidisciplinary Perspectives on Menopause**, New York: New York Academy of Sciences, 1990.

9. Reiter, RJ, **Trends in Endocrinology and Metabolism**, 1991;1:13-19.

10. Stehle JH, et al. Adrenergic signals direct rhythmic expression of transcriptional repressor CREM in the pineal gland. **Nature**, 1993;365:314-320.

11. Pearson D, Shaw S. **Life Extention**. New York: Warner Books, Inc. 1982.

12. Ganong WF, et al (eds). **The Hypothalmic-Pituitary Adrenal Axic Revisited**. New York: New York Academy of Sciences, 1987.

13. Colgan M. **Optimum Sports Nutrition.** New York: Advanced Research Press, 1993.

14. Kalimi M, Regelson W, (eds). **The Biologic Role of Dehydroepiandrosterone (DHEA)** New York: Walter de Gruyter, 1990.

Chapter 15: Estrogen Therapy

1. Longcope C. Hormone dynamics at the menopause. In Flint M, et al (eds). **Multidisciplinary Perspectives on Menopause**, New York: New York Academy of Sciences, 1990, 21-30.

2. Flint M, et al. (eds). **Multidisciplinary Perspectives on Menopause**, New York: New York Academy of Sciences, 1990.

3. **Physicians Desk Reference, 49th Edition.** Montvale NJ: Medical Economics, 1995.

4. **Time**, 26 June 1995, p. 49.

5. **Science News**, 13 May 1991.

6. Robinson RW, Lebeau RJ. Effect of conjugated equine estrogens on serum lipids and the clotting mechanism. **J Atherosci Res**, 1965;5:120-124.

7. Cauley JA, et al. Menopausal estrogen use, HDL cholesterol subfractions and liver function. **Atherosclerosis**, 1983;49:31-39.

8. Farish E, et al. The effects of conjugated equine oestrogens with and without a cyclical progestogen on lipoproteins, and HDL subfractions in postmenopausal women. **Acta Endocrinol**, 1986;113:123-127.

9. Krauss RM, et al. Effects of estrogen dose and smoking on lipid and llipoprotein levels in postmenopausal women. **Am J Obstet Gynecol**, 1988;158:1606-1611.

10. Barrett-Connor E, et al. Postmenopausal estrogen use and heart disease risk factors in the 1980s. **J Am Med Assoc**, 1989;261:2095-2100.

11. Sherwin BB, Gelfand MM. A prospective one-year study of estrogen and progestin in postmenopausal women: effects on clinical symnptoms and lipoprotein lipids. **Obstet Gynecol**, 1989;73:759-766.

12. Sonnendecker EW, et al Serum lipoprotein effects of conjugated estrogen and a sequential conjugated estrogen-medrogestone regimen in hysterectomized postmenopausal women. **Am J Obstet Guynecol**, 1989;160:1128-1134.

13. Sacks FM, et al. Low doses of postmenopausal estrogens may be optimal to favorably alter plasma lipoproteins. **Circulation**, 1989;80:329.

14. Ross RK, et al. A case-control study of menopausal estrogen therapy and breast cancer. **JAMA**, 1980;243:1635-1639.

15. Brinton LA, et al. Menopausal estrogen use and risk of breast cancer. **Cancer**, 1981;47:2517-2522.

16. Hoover R, et al. Conjugated estrogens and breast cancer risk in women. **J Natl Cancer Inst**, 1981;67:815-820.

17. Brinton LA. Menopause and risk of breast cancer. **Ann NY Acad Sci**, 1990;592:357-362.

18. Colgan M. **The New Nutrition: Medicine for the Millennium.** Vancouver: Apple Publishing, 1994.

19. Lituka H, Naito A. **Microbial Transformation of Steroids and Alkaloids.** State College, PA: University Park Press, 1967.

20. Tzingournis VA, et al. Estriol in the management of menopause. **J Amer Med Assoc**, 1978;239:1638-1641.

21. Lauritzen C. Results of a five-year prospective study of estriol succinate treatment in patients with climateric complaints. **Horm Metab Res**, 1987;19:579-584.

22. Heimer GM, Englund DE. Estriol in the treatment of postmenopausal Burogenital atrophy. **Ann NY Acad Sci**, 1990;592:428-429.

23. Guo-jun C, et al. Prospective double-blind study of CEE_3 in peri and postmenopausal women: Effects on bone loss and lipoprotein levels. **Chinese Med J**, 1994;103:929-933.

Chapter 16 Progesterone Wins

1. Metcalfe MG. Incidence of ovulation from the menarche to the menopause: observations of 622 New Zealand women. **NZ Med J,** 1983:96:645-648.

2. Lenton EA, et al. Normal variations in the length of the luteal phase: Identification of the short luteal phase. **Brit J Obstet Gynecol,** 1984;91:685-689.

3. Longcope C. Hormone dynamics at the menopause. In Flint M, et al (eds). **Multidisciplinary Perspectives on Menopause,** New York: New York Academy of Sciences, 1990;21-30.

4. **Physicians Desk Reference, 50th Edition.** Montvale NJ: Medical Economics, 1996.

5. Silfverstolpe G, et al. Lipid Metabolic studies in oophorectomized women: effects on serum lipids and lipoproteins of three synthetic progestogens. **Maturitas,** 1982;4:103-111.

6. Hirvonen E, et al. Effects of different progestogens on lipoproteins during postmenopausal replacement therapy. **N Engl J Med,** 1981; 304:560-563.

7. Ottosson UB, et al. Subfractions of high-density lipoprotein cholesterol: a comparison between progestogens and natural progesterone, **Am J Obstet Gynecol,** 1985;151:746-750.

8. Hargrove JT, et al. Menopausal hormone replacement therapy with continuous daily oral micronized estradiol and progesterone. **Obstet Gynecol,** 1989;4:606-612.

9. Meyerson B. Relationship between the anaesthetic and gestagenic action and estrus behavior inducing activity of different progestins. **Endocrinol,** 1967;81:369-374.

10. Kaness FJ, et al. Mood and behavioral changes with progestational agents. **Brit J Psychiat,** 1967;113:265-268.

11. Morrison JC, et al. the use of medroxyprogesterone acetate for rellief of climateric symptoms. **Amer J Obstet Bynecol,** 1980;138:99.

12. Backstrom T, et al. Ovarian steroid hormones: effects on mood, behavior and brain excitability. **Acta Obstet Gynacol Scand**, 1985;Suppl;130:19-24.

13. Dalton K. The premenstrual syndrom. **Brit Med J**. 1953;1:1007.

14. Moline ML. Pharmacologic strategies for managing premenstrual syndrome. **Clin Pharm**, 1993;12:181-196.

15. Lee J. **Natural Progesterone.** London: BLL Publishing, 1993.

16. Kenton L. **Passage to Power.** London: Ebury Press, 1995.

17. Lee JR. Is natural progesterone the missing link in osteoporosis prevention and treatment? **Med Hypothesis.** 1991;35:314-318.

18. Prior JC. Progesterone is a bone-trophic hormone. **Endocrine Rev;**11:386-398.

19. Colgan M. **Optimum Sports Nutrition.** New York: Advanced Research Press, 1993.

20. Rosenfeld JA. Update on continuous estrogen-progestin replacement therapy. **Amer Family Physician,** 1994;50:1519-1523.

Chapter 17. Melatonin: Top Dog

1. Reiter, RJ, **Trends in Endocrinology and Metabolism,** 1991;1:13-19.

2. Pierpaoli W, et al (eds). **The Aging Clock.** New York: New York Academy of Sciences, 1994.

3. Reiter, RJ, et al. A review of the evidence supporting melatonin's role as an antioxidant. **J Pineal Res,** 1995;18:1-11.

4. Maestroni GJ, et al. Pineal melatonin: Its fundamental immunoregulatory role in aging and cancer. **Ann NY Acad Sci,** 1988;521:140-148.

5. Dawson D, Encel N. Melatonin and sleep in humans. **J Pineal Res,** 1993;15:1-12.

6. Valcavi R, et al. Melatonin stimulates growth hormone secretion through pathways other than the growth hormone releasing hormone. **Clin Endocrinol,** 1993;39:193-199.

7. Dakshinamurti K, et al. Neurobiology of pyridoxine. **Ann NY Acad Sci,** 1990;585:128-144.

8. Colgan M. **Optimum Sports Nutrition.** New York: Advanced Research Press, 1993.

9. Colgan M. **The New Nutrition: Medicine for the Millennium.** Vancouver: Apple Publishing, 1994.

Chapter 18: Selegiline For Life

1. Dow A. **Deprenyl: The Anti-Aging Drug.** Clearwater FL: Hallberg Publishing, 1993.

2. **Physicians Desk Reference, 49th Edition.** Montvale NJ: Medical Economics, 1995.

3. **US News and World Report,** 26 June 1995, 63.

4. Knoll J. Deprenyl medication: A strategy to modulate the age-related decline of the striatal dopaminergic system. **J Am Geriat Soc,** 1992;40:839-847.

5. Schatzberg AF, Cole JO. **Manual of Clinical Pharmacology 2nd Edition.** Washington DC: American Psychiatric Press, 1990.

6. Knoll J, et al. Striatal dopamine, sexual activity, and lifespan. **Life Sciences,** 1989;45:525-531.

7. Mann J, Gershon S. Deprenyl: A selective monoamine oxidase Type-B inhibitor in endogenous depression. **Life Sci,** 1980;26:877-882.

Chapter 19 Acetyl L Carnitine

1. Taglialatela G, et al. Acetyl-L-carnitine enhances the response of Pc12 cells to nerve growth factor. **Brain Dev Res,** 1991;59:221-230.

2. Bossoni G, Carpi C. Effect of acetyl-L-carnitine on conditioned reflex learning rate and retention in laboratory animals. **Drugs Exp Clin Res,** 1986;12:911-916.

3. Ramacci MT, et al. Effect of long-term treatment with acetyl-L-carnitine on structural changes of aging rat brains. **Drugs Exp Clin Res,** 1988;14:593-601.

4. Geremia E. Antioxidant actions of acetyl-L-carnitine: In vitro study. **Med Sci Res,** 1988;16:699-700.

5. Dowson JH, et al. The morphology of lipopigment in rat purkinje neurons after chronic acetyl-L-carnitine administration. **Bid Psych Morphon,** 1992;32:179-187.

6. Malone H, et al. Altered neuro-exitability in experimental diabetic neuropathy effect of acetyl-L-carnitine. **Int J Clin Pharmacol,** 1992;12:237-241.

7. Cunti D, et al. Effect of aging and acetyl-L-carnitine on energetic and cholinergic metabolism in rat brain regions. **Mech Aging Devt,** 1989;47:39-45.

8. White HL, Scates PW. Acetyl-L-carnitine as a precursor of acetylcholine. **Neurochem Res,** 1990;15:597-601.

9. Pettigrew JW, et al. Chemical and neurochemical effects of acetyl-L-carnitine in Alzheimer's disease. **Neurobiol Aging,** 1995;16:1-4.

10. Cucinotti D, et al. Multicenter clinical placebo-controlled study with acetyl-L-carnitine in the treatment of mildly demented elderly patients. **Drug Dev Res,** 1988;14:213-216.

11. Lino A, et al. Psycho-functional changes in attention and learning under the action of L-acetylcarnitine in 17 young subjects. **Clin Ther,** 1992;140:569-543.

12. Sershen H, et al. Effect of acetyl-L-carnitine on the dopaminergic system in aging animals. **J Neurosci,** 1991;30:555-559.

13. Napoleone P, et al. Age dependent nerve cell loss in the brain of Sprogue-Dawley rats: Effect of long-term acetyl-L-carnitine treatment. **Arch Gerontal Geriat,** 1990;10:173-185.

Chapter 20: The DHEA Bandwagon

1. Barrett-Connor E, et al. A prospective study of dehydroepiandrosterone sulfate, mortality and cardiovascular disease. **New Engl J Med,** 1986;315:1519-1524.

2. Kalimi M, Regelson W, (eds). **The Biologic Role of Dehydroepiandrosterone.** New York: de Gruyter, 1990.

3. Holden C. Interest grows in anti-aging drug. **Science**, 1995;269:33.

4. Bilger B. Forever young. **Sciences**, 1995;September/October:26-31.

5. Regelson W, et al. Dehydroepiandrosterone (DHEA) "The Mother Steroid." **Ann NY Acad Sci**, 1994;719:553-563.

6. Cleary MP. Minireview. The antiobesity effect of dehydroepiandrosterone in rats. **Proc Soc Exp Biol Med**, 1991;196:8-16.

7. Cleary MP, et al. Effects of short-term dehydroepiandrosterone treatment on serum and pancreatic insulin in Zucker rats. **J Nutr**, 1988;118:382-387.

8. Berdanier CD. Dehydroepiandrosterone DHEA: useful or useless as an antiobesity agent. **Nutrition Today**, 1993;November/December: 34-38.

9. Usiskin KS, et al. Lack of effect of dehydroepiandrosterone in obese men. **Int J Obesity**, 1990;14:457-463.

10. Carlstrom KS, et al. Dehydroepiandrosterone sulfate and dehydroepiandrosterone in serum. Differences related to age and sex. **Maturitas**, 1988;10:297-306.

11. Rosenberg S, et al. Serum levels of dehydroepiandrosterone sulfate in the perimenopause. **Ann NY Acad Sci**, 1990;592:469-471.

12. Barrett-Connor E, Edelstein SL. A prospective study of dehydroepiandrosterone sulfate and cognitive function in an older population: The Rancho Bernardo Study. **J Am Geriat Soc**, 1994;42:420-423.

13. Bologna L, et al. Dehydroepiandrosterone and its sulfated derivative reduce neuronal death and enhance astrocytic differentiation in brain cell cultures. **J Neurosci Res**, 1987;17:225-234.

14. Rudman D, et al. Plasma dehydroepiandrosterone sulfate in nursing home men. **J Am Geriat Soc**, 1990;38:421-427.

15. Nasman B, et al. Serum dehydroepiandrosterone sulfate in Alzheimer's disease and in multi-infarct dementia. **Biol Psychiat**, 1991;30:684-690.

16. Helzlsover KJ, et al. Relationship of prediagnostic serum levels of dehydroepiandrosterone to the risk of developing premenopausal breast cancer. **Cancer Res**, 1992;52:1-4.

17. Cumming DC, et al. Evidence for an influence of the ovary on circulatory dehydroepiandrosterone sulfate levels. **J Clin Endocrinol Metab**, 1982;54:1069-1071.

18. Gordon GB, et al. Relationships of dehydroepiandrosterone to risk of developing postmenopausal breast cancer. **Cancer Res**, 1990;50:3859-3862.

19. Roberts E, et al. Effects of dehydroepiandrosterone and its sulfate on brain tissue in culture and on memory in mice. **Brain Res**, 1987;406:357-362.

20. Ebeling P, Koivisto VA. Physiological importance of dehydroepiandrosterone. **Lancet**, 1994;343:1479-1481.

21. Crespo D, et al. Interactions between melatonin and estradiol on morphological and morphometric features of MCF-7 human breast cancer cells. **J Pineal Res**, 1994;16:215-222.

22. Holden C. Interest grows in anti-aging drug. **Science**, 1995;269:33.

23. Barrett-Connor E, Khaw KT. Absence of an inverse relation of dehydroepiandrosterone sulfate with cardiovascular mortality in postmenopausal women. **New Engl J Med**, 1987;317:711.

24. Bush TL, et al. Cardiovascular mortality and non-contraceptive use of estrogen in women: results from the Lipid Research Clinics Program Follow-Up Study. **Circulation**, 1987;75:1102-1109.

25. Rotter JI, et al. A genetic component to the variation of dehydroepiandrosterone. **Metabolism**, 1985;34:731-736.

26. Williams DP, et al. Relationship of bodyfat percentage and fat distribution with dehydroepiandrosterone in premenopausal females. **J Clin Endocrin Metab**, 1993;77:80-85.

27. Nestler JE, et al. Dehydroepiandrosterone reduces serum low-density lipoprotein levels and bodyfat but doesn't alter insulin sensitivity in normal man. **J Clin Endocrinol Metab**, 1988;66:57-61.

28. Mortola J, Yen SSC. Effects of dehydroepiandrosterone on endocrine metabolic parameters in post-menopausal women. **J Endocrinol Metab**, 1990;71:696-704.

29. Morales A, et al. Effects of replacement dose of dehydroepiandrosterone in men and women of advancing age. **J Clin Endocrin Metab**, 1994;78:1360-1367.

30. Reaven GM, et al. Role of insulin in endogenous hypertriglyceridemia. **J Clin Invest**, 1967;46:1756-1767.

31. Sowinska-Srzednicka J, et al. Hyperinsulemia and decreased levels of dehydroepidandrosterone sulfate in premenopausal women with coronary heart disease. **J Intern Med**, 1995;237:465-472.

32. Haffner SM, et al. Decreased testosterone and dehydroepiandrosterone sulfate concentrations and associated with increased insulin and glucose concentrations in men. **Metabolism**, 1994;43:599-603.

33. Coleman DL, et al. Therapeutic effects of dehydroepiandrosterone in diabetic mice. **Diabetes**, 1982;31:830-833.

34. Coleman DL, et al. Effects of genetic background on the therapeutic effects of dehydroepiandrosterone in diabetes-obesity mutants and in aged normal mice. **Diabetes**, 1984;33:26-32.

35. Casson PR, et al. Replacement of dehydroepiandrosterone enhances T-lymphocyte insulin binding in postmenopausal women. **Fertil Steril**, 1995;63:1027-1031.

36. Fried SK, et al. Lipoprotein lipase regulation by insulin and glucocorticoid in subcutaneous and omental adipose tissues of obese women and men. **J Clin Invest**, 1993;92:2191-2198.

37. Zumoff B. Hormonal Abnormalties in Obesity. **Acta Med Scand**, 1988;723:153-160.

38. Porter JR, et al. The effect of discontinuing dehydroepiandrosterone supplementation on Zucker rat food intake and hypothalamic neurotransmitters. **Int J Obesity**, 1995;19:480-488.

39. Bremmer WJ, et al. Loss of circadian rhythmicity in blood testosterone levels with aging in normal men. **J Clin Endocrin Metab**, 1983;56:1278-1281.

Chapter 21 Growth Hormone

1. Rudman D, et al. Effects of human growth hormone in men over 60 years old. **New Engl J Med**, 1990;323:1-6.

2. Weiss R. A shot at youth. **Health,** November/December 1993;38-47.

3. Daughaday WH. The anterior pituitary. **Williams Textbook of Endocrinology**, 1985, 7th ed; 577-611.

4. Philips & Vassukopoulou-Sellin, Somatomedins; New Eng J Med, 1980;302:371-380.

5. Rudman D. Growth hormone, body composition, and aging. **J Am Geriat Soc**, 1985;33:800-807.

6. Finkelstein JW, et al. Age-related changes in the 24-hour spontaneous secretion of growth hormone. **J Clin Endocrin Metab**, 1972;35:665-670.

7. Hoffman DM, et al. Diagnosis of growth hormone deficiency in adults. **Lancet**, 1994;343:1064-1068.

8. Saini S, et al. Reproductibility of 24-hour growth-hormone profiles in man. **Clin Endocrinol**, 1991;34:455-462.

9. Hoffman DM, et al. Diagnosis of growth hormone deficiency in adults. **Lancet**, 1994;343:1064-1068.

10. Poehlman ET, Copeland KC. Influence of physical activity on insulin-like growth factor-1 in healthy younger and older men. **J Clin Endocrinol Metab,** 1990;71:1468-1473.

11. Crist DM, et al. Body composition response to exogenous GH diving training in highly conditioned athletes. **J Appl Physiol**, 1988;65:579-584.

12. **Longevity,** August 1994.

13. Yarasheski KE, Zachwieja JJ. Growth hormone therapy for the elderly. The fountain of youth proves toxic. **J Amer Med Assoc,** 1993;270:1694.

14. Snyder DK, et al. Anabolic effects of growth hormone in obese diet restricted subjects are dose dependent. **Am J Clin Nutr,** 1990;52:431-437.

15. Lehmann S, Cerra FB. Growth hormone and nutritional support - Adverse metabolic effects. **NCP,** 1992;7:27-30.

16. Ziegler TR, et al. Metabolic effects of recombinant human growth hormone in patients receiving pareneteral nutrition. **Ann Surg,** 1988;208:6-16.

17. Binnerts A, et al. The effects of human growth hormone administration in elderly adults with recent weight loss. **Clin Endocrinol Metab,** 1988;67:1312-1316.

18. Malozowski S, et al. Acute pancreatitis associated with growth hormone therapy for short stature.**New Engl J Med,** 1995;332:401-402.

19. Morales A, et al. Effects of replacement dose of dehydroepiandrosterone in men and women of advancing age. **J Clin Endocrin Metab,** 1994;78:1360-1367.

Chapter 22: Testosterone For Men

1. **Medical Tribune,** 6 August 1992.

2. **Wall Street Journal,** 3 October 1995.

3. **USA Today,** 23 May 1994.

4. Ruzicka L, Wettstein A. Uber die Krystalliche herstellung des Testikelhormons (Androsten-3-on-17-ol). **Helvetica Chimica Acta,** 1935;18:1264-1275.

5. Colgan M. Age decline of androgens in males and implications for hormone replacement therapy. **3rd International Conference on Anti-Aging and Biomedical Technology,** 1995.

6. Stokkan KA, et al. Food restriction retards aging of the pineal gland. **Brain Res,** 1991;545:66-72.

7. Smith MR, Rudd BT, Shirley A, et al. A radioimmunoassay for the estimation of serum dehydroepiandrosterone sulfate in normal and pathological sera. **Clin Chim Acta,** 1975;65:5.

8. Orentreich N, Brind JL, Rizer RL, Vogelman JH. Age changes and sex differences in serum dehydroepiandrosterone sulfate concentrations throughout adulthood. **J Clin Endocrinol Metab,** 1984;59:551-555.

9. Warner BA, Dufan ML, Santen RL. Effects of aging and illness on the pituitary testicular axis in men: Qualitative as well as quantitative changes in luteinizing hormone. **J Clin Endocrinol Metab,** 1985;60:263-268.

10. Tenover JS, Dahl KD, Hsueh AJW, Lim P, Matsumoto AM, Bremmer WJ. Serum bioactive and immunoreactive follicle-stimulating

hormone levels and the response to clomiphene in healthy young and elderly men. **J Clin Endocrinol Metab**, 1986;64:1103-1108.

11. Vekemans M, Robyn C. Influence of age on serum prolactin levels in women and men. **Br J Med**, 1975;27:738-739.

12. Salem SI, et al. Response of the reproductive system of male rats to protein and zinc deficiency during puberty. **Ann Nutr Metab**, 1984;28:44.

13. Abbassi AA, et al Experimental zinc deficiency in man. Effect on testicular function. **J Lab Clin Med**, 1980;96:544.

14. Colgan M. **Optimum Sports Nutrition**. New York, NY: Advanced Research Press, 1993.

15. World Health Organization Task Force on Methods for the Regulation of Male Fertility, Contraceptive efficacy of testosterone-induced azoospermia in normal men, **Lancet**, 1990;336:955-959.

16. Humbert W, Pevet P, In Pierpaoli W, et al (eds). **The Aging Clock**, New York: New York Academy of Sciences, 1994;43.

17. Knoll J. Deprenyl medication: A strategy to modulate the age-related decline of the striatal dopaminergic system. **J Am Geriat Soc**, 1992;40:839-847.

18. Kalimi M, Regelson W (eds). **The Biologic Role of Dehydroepiandrosterone**, New York; de Guyter Publishing, 1990.

19. Colgan M. **The New Nutrition: Medicine for the Millennium**. Vancouver: Apple Publishing, 1994.

20. Vermeulen A, Kaufman JM. Aging of the hypothalamo-pituitary-testicular axis in men. **Horm Res**. 1995;43:25-28.

21. Yesalis CE, (ed). **Anabolic Steroids in Sport and Exercise**. Champaign, IL: Human Kinetics, 1993.

22. Taylor WN. **Anabolic Steroids and The Athlete**. London: McFarland and Co, 1982.

23. **Physicians Desk Reference, 49th Edition.** Montvale NJ: Medical Economics, 1995, p. 1144.

24. World Health Organization. Contraceptive efficiency of testosterone-induced azoospermia in normal men. **Lancet**, 1990;336:955-959.

25. Brown-Sequard CE. Des effects produits chez l'homme d'un liquide retire des testicules frais de cobaye et de chien. **CR Soc Biol (Paris)**, 1889;1:420-430.

26. Conway AJ, et al. Randomized clinical trial of testosterone replacement in hypogonadal men. **Internat J Androl**, 1988;11:247-264.

27. Place VA, et al. Transdermal testosterone replacement through genital skin. Nieschlog E, Behr HM (Eds). **Testosterone: Action, Deficiency, Substitution**. New York: Springer-Verlag 1990.

28. Cunningham GR, et al. Testosterone replacement with transdermal therapeutic systems. **J Amer Med Assoc**, 1989;261:2525-2530.

29. Bremmer WJ, et al. Loss of circadian rhythmicity in blood testosterone levels with aging in normal men. **J Clin Endocrin Metab**, 1983;56:1278-1281.

30. American Hospital Formilary Service Product Information for the Testoderm Testosterone Transdermal System. American Society of Hospital Pharmacists, 1985.

Chapter 23: Testosterone for Women

1. Longcope C, et al. Steroid and gonadotropin levels in women during the peri-menopausal years, **Maturitas**, 1986;8:189-196.

2. Longcope C. Adrenal and gonadal androgen secretion in normal females. **Clin Endocrinol Metab**, 1986;15:213-228.

3. Rannevik G, et al. A prospective long-term study in women from pre-menopause to post-menopause: Changing profiles of gonadotropins, oestrogens and androgens. **Maturitas**, 1986;8:297-307.

4. Poortman J, et al. Adrenal androgen secretion and metabolism in postmenopausal women. In Gemazzini AR, et al (eds). **Adrenal Androgens** New York:Rowen Press;1980:219-240.

5. Sherwin BB. Affective changes with estrogen and androgen replacement therapy in surgically menopausal women. **J Affective Dis**, 1988;14:177-187.

6. Sherwin BB, et al. Androgen enhances sexual motivation in females: A prospective cross-over study of sex hormone administration in the surgical menopause. **Am J Obstet Gynecol**, 1985;151:153-160.

7. Sherwin BB. The role of androgens in menopausal women. In Speroff L (ed), **Androgens in the Menopause.** Proceedings of the Reid-Rowell Symposium, Atlanta, March 1988.

8. Brincat M, et al. Subcutaneous hormone implants for the control of climateric symptoms. **Lancet,** 1984;1:16-18.

9. Hazzard WR, et al. Kinetic studies on the modulation of high-density lipoprotein, apolipoprotein and subfraction metabolism by sex steroids in postmenopausal women. **Metabolism,** 1984;33:779-785.

10. Wagner JD, Paper presented to the meeting of the American College of Obstetricians and Gynecologists, San Francisco, May, 1995.

11. Sherwin BB, et al. Postmenopausal estrogen and androgen replacement and lipoprotein lipid concentration. **Am J Obstet Gynecol,** 1987;156:414-419.

12. Burger HG, et al. The management of persistent symptoms with estradiol-testosterone implants. Clinical, lipid and hormonal results. **Maturitas,** 1984;6:351-358.

13. Morell V, Zeroing in on how hormones affect the immune system. **Science,** 1995;269:773-775.

14. **Physicians Desk Reference, 35th Edition.** Montvale NJ: Medical Economics, 1981.

15. **Physicians Desk Reference, 50th Edition.** Montvale NJ: Medical Economics, 1996.

16. Personal communication with Solvay Pharmaceuticals, supplier of Estratest, 1 March 1996.

17. Buster JE, Postmenopausal steroid replacement with micronized dehydroepiandrosterone: preliminary oral bioavailability and dose proportionality studies. **Am J Obstet Gynecol,** 1992;166:1163-1170.

18. Yen S, Jaffee R. **Reproductive Endocrinology.** Philadelphia: WB Saunders, 1978.

19. Inaudi P, et al. Gonadotropin prolactin and thyrotropin secretion after exogenous dehydroepiandrostrone sulfate administration in normal women. **Horm Res,**1991;35:40.

Chapter 24 Hormonal Nutrition

1. Miguel J, et al (eds). **Handbook of Free Radicals and Antioxidants.** Boca Raton FL: CRC Press, 1989.

2. National Research Council. **Recommended Dietary Allowances, 7th ed.,** Washington, DC: National Academy Press, 1968.

3. National Research Council. **Recommended Dietary Allowances, 9th ed.,** Washington, DC: National Academy Press, 1980.

4. National Research Council. **Recommended Dietary Allowances, 10th ed.,** Washington, DC: National Academy Press, 1989.

5. Colgan M. **The New Nutrition: Medicine for the Millennium** Vancouver: Apple Publishing, 1994.

6. Colgan M. **Optimum Sports Nutrition.** New York: Advanced Research Press, 1993.

7. Colgan M. **Your Personal Vitamin Profile.** New York: William Morrow, 1982.

8. Goode HF. The effect of dietary vitamin E deficiency on plasma, zinc and copper concentrations. **Clin Nutr,** 1991;10:233-235.

9. United States Department of Agriculture. **Food Technology,** 1981;35:9.

10. Levander OA, Chengh (eds). **Micronutrient Interactions**. New York: New York Academy of Sciences, 1980.

11. Anggard E. Nitric oxide: mediator, murderer, and medicine. **Lancet,** 1994;343:1199-1207.

12. Yallampa C, et al. Steroid hormones modulate the production of nitric oxide and GMP in the rat uterus **Endocrinol** 1994;134:1971-1974.

13. Page MD, et al. Growth hormone responses to L-arginine and L-dopa alone and after GHRH pre-treatment **Clin Endocrinol.**1988;28:551-558.

14. Giustina A, et al. Arginine blocks the inhibitory effects of hydrocortisone on circulating growth hormone in patients with acromegaly. **Metabolism,**1993;42:664-668.

15. Flyvbjerg A. evidence that potassium deficiency induces growth retardation through reduced circulating levels of growth hormone and insulin like growth factor-1. **Metabolism,** 1991;40:769-775.

16. Sanchez-Capelo A, et al. Potassium regulates plasma testosterone and renal ornithine decarboxylase in mice. **FEBS Lett,** 1993;333:32-34.

17. Holden JM, et al. Zinc and copper in self-selected diets. **J Am Dietet Assoc.** 1979;75:23-28.

18. Netter A, et al. Effects of zinc administration on plasma testosterone dimydrotesterone and sperm count. **Arch Androl** 1981;7:69.

19. Hunt CD, et al. Effects of dietary zinc depletion on seminal volume and zinc loss, serum testosterone concentrations and sperm morphology in young men. **Am J Clin Nutr,** 1992;56:148-157.

20. Mertz W (ed). **Trace Elements in Human and Animal Nutrition Fifth Edition.**

21. Nestler JE, et al. Effects of insulin reduction with benfluorex or serum dehydroepiandrosterone (DHEA) DHEA sulfate and blood pressure in hypertensive middle-aged and elderly men. **J Clin Endocrinol Metab** 1995;80:700-706.

22. Nielsen FH, et al. Effect of dietary boron on mineral, estrogen and testosterone metabolism **FASEBJ,**1987;1:394-397.

23. Fernando A, Green NR. The effect of boron supplementation on lean body mass, plasma testosterone levels and strength in male weightlifters **FASEBJ,**1992;6:A1946.

24. Nielsen FH, et al. Boron enhances and mimics some effects of estrogen therapy in postmenopausal women. **J Trace Elem Exp Med,**1992;5:237-246.

25. Sachse G, Williams B. Efficiency of thiotic acid in the therapy of peripheral diabetic neuropathy. **Horm Metab Res,** 1980, Suppl 9.

26. Packer L, et al. Lipoic acid as a biological antioxidant. **Free Rad Biol Med,** 1995;19:227-250.

27. Sun AY, Sun GH. Neurochemical aspects of the membrane hypothesis of aging. **Interdiscp Topics Gerontol**, 1979;15:34-53.

28. Schroeder F. Role of lipid membrane asymmetry in aging. **Neurobiol Aging**, 1984;5:323-333.

29. Nolan KA, Blass JP. Preventing cognitive decline. **Clin Geriat**, 1992:8:19-34.

30. Bartus RT, et al. The cholinergic hypothesis of geriatric memory dysfunction. Science, 1982;217:408-417.

31. Ginidin J. The effect of plant phosphatidylserine on age associated memory impairment and mood in the functioning elderly. **Gerontologist**, 1993;33:Abstract.

32. Double-blind crossover study of phosphatidylserine vs placebo in patients with early dementia of the Alzheimer's type. **Eur Neuropsychopharmacol**, 1992;2:149-155.

33. Crook TH, et al. Effects of phosphatidylserine in age associated memory impairment. **Neurol**, 1991;41:644-649.

34. Heiss WD, et al. Long-term effects of phosphatidylserine, pyritinol and cognitive training in Alzheimer's disease. **Dementia**, 1994;5:88-98.

35. Ammasari-Teule M, et al. Chronic administration of phosphatidylserine during ontogeny enhances subject environment interactions and radial maze performance in C57/B46 mice. Physiol Behav, 1990;47:755-760.

36. 10th Annual Meeting of the American College of Clinical Gerontology, San Antonio, Texas, October 1995.

37. Centers for Disease Control. MMWR. Sheigella sonnei outbreak associated with contaminated drinking water. **J Amer Med Assoc**. 1996;275:1071.

Chapter 25 Hormonal Exercise

1. Bortz W, **J Amer Med Assoc**, 1982;248:1203-1208.

2. Colgan M. **Optimum Sports Nutrition.** New York: Advanced Research Press, 1993.

3. Colgan M. **The New Nutrition: Medicine for the Millennium.** Vancouver: Apple Publishing, 1994.

4. Blair SN, et al. **J Amer Med Assoc**, 1989;262:2395-2401.

5. National Research Council. **Recommended Dietary Allowances, 10th ed.**, Washington, DC: National Academy Press, 1989.

6. Rambout PC, Goode AW. **Lancet**, 1985;2:1050-1052.

7. Lane N, et al. **Med Sci Sports Exer**, 1988;20(S):551.

8. Smith EL, Gilligan C. **Physician Sportsmed**, 1987;15:91-100.

9. Smith EL, et al. **Calcified Tissue Intern**, 1984;36(S):129.

10. Larson L. **Acta Physiol Scand**, 1978;36(S):457.

11. **Muscular Development**, September 1995, 36.

12. McCartney NA, et al. **Amer J Cardiol**, 1991;67:939.

13. Joyce JN, et al. Age related regional loss of caudateputamen dopamine receptors revealed by quantitative radiography. **Brain Res**, 1986;378:158-163.

14. de Castro JM, et al. Operationally conditioned running: effects on brain catecholamine concentration and receptor densities in the rat. **Pharmacol Biochem Behav**, 1985;23:495-500.

15. MacRae PG, et al. Endurance training effects on striatal D2 dopamine receptor bin and striatal dopamine metabolite levels. **Neurosci Lett**, 1987;79:138-144.

16. Wang HY, et al. Exercise reduces age dependent decrease in platelet protein kinase C activity and translocation. **J Gerontol**, 1995;50A:M12-M16.

17. Poehlman ET, Copeland KC. Influence of physical activity on insulin-like growth factor-1 in healthy younger and older men. **J Clin Endocrinol Metab**, 1990;71:1468-1473.

18. Craig BW, et al. Effects of progressive resistance training on growth hormone and testosterone levels in young and elderly men. **Mech Aging Devt**, 1989;49:159-169.

19. Kraemer WJ, et al. Endogenous anabolic hormonal and growth factor responses to heavy resistance exercise in males and females. **Int J Sports Med**, 1991;12:228-235.

20. Swerdloff RS, Wang C. Androgens and aging in men. **Exper Gerontol**, 1993;28:435-446.

21. Griffith RO, et al., Testicular function during exhaustive endurance training. **Physician Sportsmed**, 1990;18:54-64.

22. Desai KM, et al. Hazards of long distance cycling **Brit Med J**, 1989;298:1072-1073.

23. Wheeler GD, et al. Endurance training decreases testosterone levels in men without change in luteinizing hormone. **J Clin Endocrinol Metab**, 1991;42:422-425.

24. Shangold M. Evaluation and management of menstrual dysfunction in athletes. **J Amer Med Assoc**, 1990;263:16665-1669.

25. **Men's Journal**, Sept. 1993, 134.

26. Notolovitz M. In Shangold M, Mirken G (eds). **Women and Exercise**, Philadelphia, PA:FA Davis, 1988.

27. **Amer J Epidemiol**, 1991;134:220.

28. **Med Sci Sports Exer**, 1992;24:714.

29. **Phychosomatics**, 1990;3:112.

30. Snyder SH, Opiate receptors in the brain. **New Engl J Med**, 1977;296:266-271.

31. Colgan M. **The Power Program.** San Diego: CI Publications, 1989.

Index

A

E

F

G

Kidney 229
Kinsey Reports 6, 23
Kirby, Dr. Roger 56
Koll, Dr. Joseph 169
Kraemer, Dr. Bill 245-246
Krug, Dr. Rosemarie 62

L

L-arginine 220, 227-228
Lancet 219
Lauerson, Dr. Neils 89, 90
L-carnitine 171, 220
L-dopa 165
Lean mass 191
Lee, Dr. John 153
Leiden University 94
Leisure World 38
Levonorgestrel 150, 151
Leydig cells 20, 62
Libido 2, 7, 10,16, 18, 20, 22, 23-24,
    47-50, 53, 54, 56-61, 72, 74, 76,
    92, 94, 103, 170, 198
Lind, Dr. James 218
Lindgren, Dr. R. 115
Lindheim, Dr. S. 112
Lindsay, Dr. Robert 109, 110
Linoleic acid 232, 234
Linopiridine 176
Lipofuscin 172
Lipogen Company 235
Lipoic acid (see alpha lipoic acid)
Liver 188, 191, 204
Longcope, Dr. Christopher 51, 149,
    210
Love, Dr. Susan 137
Low acid foods 236-238
Lupus erythymatosis 214
Luteinizing hormone 20, 22, 58,
    61, 62, 124, 200, 217

M

Manson, Dr. J 112
Masters and Johnson 6
Maturitas 115
Mayo Clinic 87, 89
McCartney, Dr. Neil 243
McCurry, Michael 243
McGill University 34, 53, 74
McMaster University, Ontario 243
Medical College of Pennsylvania
    244
Medical College of Virginia 180
Medical College of Wisconsin 191
Medical University of Lubeck 62
Medroxyprogesterone 151, 152
Melatonin 124, 127-128, 159-164,
    172, 176, 180, 184, 189, 200, 202,
    217, 231, 259
Memory 174, 183, 225, 235, 244
Menometrorrhagia 87
Menopause 9, 34, 36, 39, 44, 51,
    52, 54, 124, 132, 137, 140,
    145, 146, 149, 157, 210, 246
Menstrual cycle 149, 152, 157
Mertz, Dr. Walter 229
Methyltestosterone 204, 205, 215
Metpath Laboratories 190
Micronized progesterone 156-157
Miller, Dr. Norman 86
Minerals 162-163, 203, 219-231,
    241,   258, 259
Miscarriages 153
Mistletoe 154
Molybdenum 219
Monoamine oxidase (MAO)
    inhibitors 59, 167-168
Morales, Dr. Arlene 186
Mt Sinai School of Medicine 23

R

U

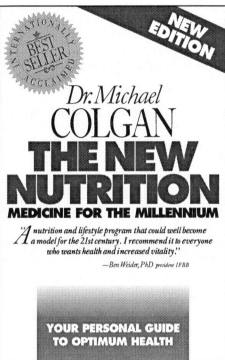
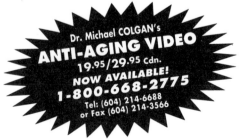